How To Treat Yourself With CHINESE HERBS

ABOUT THE AUTHOR

Dr. Hong-yen Hsu (1917–1991) was a distinguished researcher and educator. After graduating from Meiji Pharmaceutical College and the Pharmacognosy Department of Tokyo University, Dr. Hsu earned his doctorate in pharmacy at the University of Kyoto. He remained in Japan for three more years as a member of the research staff of the Department of Pharmaceutical Sciences at the University of Tokyo, before returning to Taiwan in 1945. He then became actively engaged in teaching and conducting research at National Taiwan University and medical colleges in Taipei, Taichung, and Kaohsiung. Dr. Hsu was dean of the Botany Department at the College of Chinese Culture, director of the Institute of Pharmacological Sciences at China Medical College, and president of the Oriental Healing Arts Institute. A prolific author, he published more than 100 articles in Chinese and English, and more than 30 books.

How To Treat Yourself With CHINESE HERBS

Dr. Hong-Yen Hsu

Keats Publishing, Inc. New Canaan, Connecticut

Oriental Healing Long Beach, California
Arts Institute

NOTICE

Information compiled from traditional medical texts and from the observations of modern authorities on Chinese medicine is presented here for its educational value and should not be used for treatment or prevention of disease without the advice of a Chinese physician or other medical authority.

Copyright © 1980 by Hong-yen Hsu, 1993 by Oriental Healing Arts Institute

Keats Publishing Edition published by arrangement with the Oriental Healing Arts Institute, Long Beach, California

Library of Congress Cataloging-in-Publication Data:

Hong-yen Hsu
      How to treat yourself with Chinese Herbs.
Includes index.
      1. Therapeutics. 2. Herbs—Therapeutic use. 3. Medicine,
   Chinese—Formulae, receipts, prescriptions.
1. Title.
      RM 121.H88   615′.321   78-26617
ISBN 0-87983-603-2

Printed in the United States of America

Published by Keats Publishing, Inc.
27 Pine Street (Box 876)
New Canaan, Connecticut 06840-0876

10   9   8   7   6

CONTENTS

PART I

Differentiation of Illnesses and Chinese Herbal
Formulas Appropriate for Their Treatment

PART II
A Discussion of Commonly Used
Herbal Formulas

PART III
Some Commonly Used Chinese Herbs

PART IV
Diagnostic Outlines for the 13 Most Commonly
Used Chinese Formulas

PREFACE

Technological advances have brought comfort and convenience, as well as unforeseen harm to human health in the form of environmental pollution, food adulteration, and drug toxicities. As the former director of the Bureau of Food and Drug Control of the National Health Administration for the Republic of China, I gained firsthand knowledge of the magnitude of these problems.

One of the dire consequences of industrial development and urban modernization is pollution in its myriad of forms. Factories spew out poisonous cyanides and mercurides, automobiles discharge carbon monoxide, and tens of thousands of other hazardous chemicals pervade our daily lives.

Artificial coloring, preservatives, and sweeteners, antioxidants, fungicides, and insecticides contaminate the food we eat, while giving it a longer shelf life and making it more pleasing to the eye. Excess amounts of some of these foreign substances are removed from the body by the liver, kidneys, and other organs. In healthy persons, this elimination takes place without much difficulty, though, in those who are frail or otherwise impaired, this extra burden on the body can cause exhaustion and injury.

Lastly, the widespread use of Western pharmaceuticals is primarily responsible for drug toxicities. Though they are generally quite effective at treating the targeted disease, Western therapies pose the very real risk of harmful side effects incurred by extensive or long-term use.

Chinese medicine cannot correct the ills which besiege the body due to environmental pollution and food adulteration, but it does offer an alternative to the potentially toxic side effects of Western drugs. For the most part, the herbs used in Chinese medicinal formulas are natural products similar to our daily food. Platycodon, for example, is both a cough medicine and an ingredient in Korean cuisine. For thousands of years, Chinese physicians have prescribed natural drugs, which, with very few exceptions, are nontoxic and entirely suitable for human use.

This book was written for laypersons who wish to take a more active role in their own health maintenance and in the treatment of their illnesses. Listed here are commonly used formulas for common disorders. As Chinese medicine stresses "treatment by conformation" (symptom complexes), readers may design their own treatment using this handbook as a user-friendly guide, without even knowing the name of their particular ailment. Of course, should the condition persist or worsen, a Chinese physician or other health-care professional should be consulted.

FOREWORD

The recent passing of Dr. Hong-yen Hsu, the author of *How to Treat Yourself with Chinese Herbs,* has left a void in the authoritative advocacy of Chinese herbal medicine, particularly in the United States. I first met this wonderful man in Taiwan, where I found him to be an extremely knowledgeable scientist, whose name was a household word in that country, embodying the concepts of truth, knowledge, generosity, experience, honesty and respect. Since that time I frequently met Dr. Hsu at international and national congresses and came to know his impact on Chinese herbal medicine in this country through the many books that he and his coworkers have published in this field. His writings are based on personal experience, a full knowledge of the Chinese theories of traditional medicine, an application of Western scientific principles and an ability to communicate this complex area of medicine and science.

My own initiation to the value of Chinese traditional medicine came as a result of being selected as a member of former President Richard Nixon's third exchange delegation to the People's Republic of China in 1974, covering the subject of "Herbal Pharmacology." In 26 days we analyzed information based on visits to about 20 different research institutes and hospitals, many of which were using and/or studying Chinese herbal medicine. Several physicians were members of our delegation and I believe it is safe to say that they also were impressed with what they saw. Since 1974 I have watched the scientific (Western-style) evaluation of many of the herbal medicines that we saw being used and, in most cases, a good rationale for their use, based on chemistry, pharmacology and clinical studies has come to light.

How to Treat Yourself with Chinese Herbs is now in its fifth printing and it is a tribute to the fine contributions of Dr. Hsu. The book will forever be a reminder of his ultimate goal in life, i.e., to bring to people his beliefs and thoughts on the maintenance of good health through the use of Chinese herbs. This book is simple to use, allows those who do not completely understand the theories of Chinese traditional medicine to utilize it through simplified analogies, provides cautions concerning potential side effects, and delineates the therapeutic applications of single herbs and compound mixtures.

I am happy to provide this foreword to *How to Treat Yourself with Chinese Herbs,* not only because of my friendship with and admiration of Dr. Hong-yen Hsu, but because of my interest and belief in the value of Chinese herbal medicines.

Norman R. Farnsworth, Ph.D.
Research Professor of Pharmacognosy
  and Senior University Scholar Program
  for Collaborative Research in the
  Pharmaceutical Sciences
College of Pharmacy
University of Illinois at Chicago
Chicago, Illinois   March, 1993

INTRODUCTION TO THE FIFTH PRINTING

When this book was first published in 1976, there were no licensed acupuncturists in the United States and virtually no one who could prescribe Chinese herbs, other than a few traditional Chinese doctors working secretively with Chinese immigrants as their patients. Dr. Hong-yen Hsu, the world's foremost expert in Chinese medicine as practiced in Japan and Taiwan, realized the vast potential health benefit of this medical system and wanted Westerners to be able to take advantage of it. Therefore, he wrote a book about how to treat oneself with Chinese herbs.

The process of selecting a formula for one's own use is similar to that which a well-trained practitioner uses, but one usually lacks the experience of the practitioner, while having a better insight into one's own life. To make up for the lack of medical experience, one must rely on herbal prescriptions for which a large amount of accumulated knowledge has been derived from the experience of many doctors. This book contains 113 formulas that have been used for a century or more—in most cases for 10 centuries or more. The range of applications, the safety, and the effectiveness of the formulas is well-established in the minds of practitioners who have spent years studying the subject. These formulas are taught as a standard part of the training of doctors in the Orient who prescribe Chinese herbs.

To pick a formula from the collection, one must match the formula pattern to the body pattern rather than simply looking up disease or symptom names. Formula patterns, called conformations, are revealed in the repetition of certain combinations of herbs within the prescriptions. For example:

- Ginger, jujube, and licorice (or any two of these together), are typically used in formulas intended for quick action in the treatment of acute ailments. Their function is to promote the function of the digestive system and hence nourish the healing energies of the body.

- Coptis and scute (sometimes with phellodendron and/or gardenia) are typically used in formulas to relieve inflammation. They might be used, for example, to treat skin eruptions, sore throat, or irritated intestines.

- Hoelen and alisma (sometimes with atractylodes and/or magnolia bark) are typically used in formulas to get rid of accumulated moisture. The accumulation may show up as edema or in the digestive system with abdominal bloating or diarrhea.

- Cardamon and saussurea (sometimes with ginger) are used to treat pain, usually in the chest or abdomen. These spicy herbs break up congestion of the circulation that can lead to sensation of pain.

- Bupleurum and pinellia (sometimes with scute, ginger, or citrus) are used in harmonizing formulas. These usually treat syndromes that involve nervousness, stress, muscle tension, and digestive irregularities. The herbs also reduce inflammation of internal organs, such as the liver.

- Cinnamon and peony are used to relax the muscles and promote the circulation of blood. They also help treat the early stage of illnesses.

- Aconite and cinnamon (and sometimes atractylodes) are used to treat chilly symptoms that usually produce aching in the back or limbs.

- Ginseng and licorice are used to strengthen vitality, improve digestion, and assist homeostatic mechanisms.

- Tang-kuei and peony (sometimes with rehmannia and/or cnidium) are used to nourish the blood and regulate menstruation.

- Platycodon and fritillaria (and sometimes morus and/or apricot seed) are used to relieve coughing and resolve lung diseases.

- Ma-huang and licorice (sometimes with apricot seed, cinnamon, gypsum, or ginger) are used to relieve acute respiratory disorders and to induce perspiration.

- Siler and angelica (sometimes with chiang-huo, mentha, or schizonepeta) are used to relieve pain in the skin and muscles or inflammation affecting the surface portions of the body: skin, sinuses, eyes, nose, throat.

- Rhubarb and linum (sometimes with magnolia bark and chih-chih) are used to resolve constipation.

These are just a few examples of the component parts of formulas found in this book. When the herbs are combined into complete prescriptions—usually containing from three to ten herbs—they aim like an arrow at patterns of disharmony that have been recognized by Chinese doctors. These unhealthy patterns that lead to disease or discomfort are often quickly dissipated by consuming the herbs in the proper dosage, allowing the body to restore its basic balance. It took the wisdom of the best doctors, and the continual evolution of this medical field, to determine which patterns tended to go together and therefore which herbs must be brought into the same tea or pill to yield the desired effects.

While the 113 formulas are not intended for use in resolving serious diseases by themselves, they can play a part in helping the body to heal. Hence, for example, the famous Rehmannia Six Formula and Rehmannia Eight Formula (which differs from the former by the addition of cinnamon and aconite), are used today in Japan and China for some patients suffering from hypertension, kidney stones, cataracts, cancer, back pain, diabetes, or premature aging. The wide range of applications comes from the Chinese theory that many different diseases can arise from an imbalance of certain organ systems; these two formulas are known to be effective in treating a "deficiency syndrome" that is associated with the "kidney system."

The secondary effects of the formulas include balancing of hormones, regulation of blood components, and improvement of immune functions. Similarly, Ginseng and Astragalus combination and Minor Bupleurum combination are widely used formulas that have been applied in the treatment of hepatitis, colitis, AIDS, chronic bronchitis, diarrhea, and stress-induced ulcer. Both formulas treat a "deficiency syndrome" associated with the "spleen system." The secondary effects of the formulas include reduction of inflammation, normalization of immune responses, and improvements of digestive functions. As it turns out, modern drugs do a reasonably good job of treating simple "excess syndromes," because they usually have the effect of inhibiting a physiologic function, including its pathological aspects, but Chinese herb formulas are important for the resolution of "deficiency syndromes," because they can promote physiologic functions.

At this time, nearly 20 years after the first English-language edition of this book was published, one need not rely only on self-treatment with Chinese herbs. There are now thousands of licensed acupuncturists working throughout the United States, many of whom are trained to prescribe Chinese herbs. In addition, several other health professionals, notably naturopathic physicians, but also chiropractors, medical doctors, and massage therapists, have also obtained some training in this field. Therefore, for more serious ailments, one can consult these professionals in order to obtain a completely therapeutic program that will include Chinese herbs.

Whether you use this book to self-select formulas or to better understand the formulas prescribed to you, it is a rich resource. My own studies of this book stimulated me to begin teaching, in 1980, about traditional Chinese herb formulas to students who were mainly pursuing a study of Western herbs; this was a shift away from simply describing the use of individual Chinese or Western herbs. From those early classes I developed a text, *Chinese Herbology,* which has served as an advanced training program for acupuncturists and others interested in the field for the past decade. One of the points made in that program, as well as elsewhere in my own work, is that one cannot gain a firm grasp of Chinese medicine without knowing about—and understanding—the basic formulas from which doctors in China (and throughout the Orient) have gained extensive experience. These formulas are presented in *How to Treat Yourself with Chinese Herbs*.

For those who find this book of value and wish to pursue the subject further, Dr. Hsu has written a more comprehensive text (which was recently revised): *Commonly Used Chinese Herb Formulas with Illustrations*. It expands the number of herb formulas to nearly 400 and divides them by therapeutic categories. In addition, Dr. Hsu and his colleagues have produced two dozen other books on a vast array of subjects related to Chinese medicine to provide a comprehensive look at the field.

Subhuti Dharmananda, Ph.D.
Director, Institute for Traditional Medicine
Portland, Oregon   February, 1993

A BRIEF INTRODUCTION
TO CHINESE HERBS

In China and Southeast Asia, diseases are treated by Western as well as Chinese therapies. Western therapy adopts an objective approach which first establishes the name of the disease, or the "heteropathy," and then prescribes treatment specific to that disease. Chinese therapy, however, gives special attention to the patient's pains, or the "conformation," and can prescribe a general treatment on a subjective basis before even identifying the disease by name. Western medicine emphasizes diagnosis, while Chinese medicine emphasizes treatment. Although both of them aim to alleviate pain, their theories and therapies vary considerably. The former uses mainly purified chemicals, while the latter employs various herbs and natural materials.

Chinese medical theory is based on two written works, *Shang Han Lun* (Treatise on Diseases and Fevers) and *Chin Kuei Yao Lueh* (Summaries of Household Treatments) by CHANG Chung Ching. This empirical system has been followed very effectively in countless human cases throughout the past 2,000 years. There were some supplements in later generations, but no objections or proposals of abandonment have ever been suggested.

Characteristic of Chinese medicine is observation of the patient's personal constitution and consideration of his heredity, environment, and the way in which his disease developed. All of these factors indicate various conformations. The conformations are generally divided into "Eight Principles" and "Six Stages." Herbal formulas are then administered according to the confirmation instead of the disease name.

The Eight Principles are the external environmental factors,

RIGHT—Chang Chung-Ching, A.D. 142-220, probably the world's first medical specialist, established the Chinese formula therapy during the Latter Han Dynasty. From his portrait in the collection of the Imperial Palace.

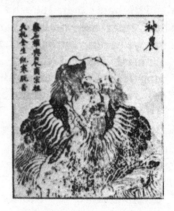

LEFT—From Chang's book, *On Typhoid.*

RIGHT—Sheng Nung, c. 3494 B.C., I is the Chinese God of Husbandry. From a wood carving.
(Also Shen Nung.)

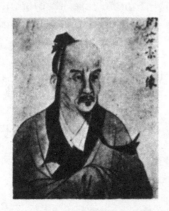

LEFT—Tao-Hung-Ching, A.D. 452-536, collected ancient records for *The Book on Herbs by Sheng Nung.* His greatest contribution was his study of herbs.

namely: yin, yang, weakness, firmness, surface, inside, chill, and heat. According to observation of the "confirmation," treatment consists of natural herbal formulas with contrasting natures. For example, Panax ginseng, Angelicae Radix, and similar herbs are used to supplement the weak physique; Coptidis Rhizoma and others are used to dispel heat in diseases with fever. All promote equilibrium of the physical condition and maximum health.

The *Shan Han Lun* also divides the progress of disease into six phases (known as the "Six Stages" in Chinese medicine) as follows:

Yang (Positive) Diseases

Greater Yang Disease: The main symptoms are floating pulse, headache, fever, and severe chills.

Lesser Yang Disease: The main symptoms are bitter taste in the mouth, dry throat, dizziness, and vomiting.

Sunlight Yang Disease: There are stomach and abdominal symptoms accompanied by severe chills and constipation or diarrhea.

Yin (Negative) Disease

Greater Yin Disease: The main symptoms are diarrhea, vomiting, and dysentery.

Lesser Yin Disease: The main symptoms are sinking pulse, severe chills, fatigue, and cold hands and feet.

Absolute Yin Disease: The main symptoms are thirst, oliguria, and exhaustion.

There are appropriate herb formulas to match and treat each of the above six phases.

In the establishment of conformation in Chinese medicine, there is a particular diagnostic approach encompassing four methods. These are as follows:

Visual Observation: In this method the eyes are used to observe the physical structure, complexion, skin color, nails, eyes, and dryness of the skin. For example, the physically strong and well-nourished generally belong to the firm confirmation; on the other hand, the physically lean who are pale and have a delicate bone structure with flaccid muscles belong to the weak conformation.

Observation by Hearing and Smelling: In this method the sense of hearing is used to listen for coughs, stridor, and number and quality of respirations; the sense of smell is used to identify odors of the mouth and body.

Questioning: This method is used when asking about the patient's subjective complaints such as fever, perspiration, severe or mild chills, thirst, dryness of throat, headache, dizziness, tinnitus, difficulty with elimination, vomiting, abdominal aches, chest pain, edema, appetite, and other symptoms.

Palpation: In this method the sense of touch is used to feel the pulse and the condition of the abdomen. In feeling the pulse, it should be noted if it is sinking, late, fast, long, short, or tense. This is done in order to identify the patient's surface, inside, weak, firm, chill, and fever confirmations. Abdominal palpation means feeling the abdomen of the patient in order to determine his weakness or firmness by the elasticity and reaction of the skin. In conjunction with the patient's history, the above diagnoses are a basis on which treatment may be prescribed.

Shan Ching (The Classic on the Mountain, 250 B.C.) and *Hai-Ching* (The Classic on the Sea, 120 B.C.) first recorded 68 effective drugs of plant and animal origin, such as Cinnamomi Ramulus, Rhei Rhizoma, and talcum, which have been widely used up to the present time. However, it has been generally recognized that the first classic was *Shen Nung Pen Tsao Ching* (Shen Nung's Classic of Herbs) of about A.D. 25. It has been said that Shen Nung taught the people to till the land. He also personally tasted various kinds of herbs. Although later fatally poisoned by a toxic herb, he left behind much valuable research. TAO Hung Ching (about A.D. 502) revised Shen Nung's work into a commentary that comprises 365 varieties of superior, general, and inferior herb drugs. These categories are described as follows:

Superior herb drugs: Imperial herbs or tonics that may be taken for a long duration. They include Glycyrrhizae Radix,

Panax Ginseng, Bupleuri Radix, and Cinnamomi Radix.

General herb drugs: Ministerial herbs or nutrients that may be used to treat diseases. They include Zingiberis Rhizoma, Angelicae Sinensis Radix, and Ephedrae Radix.

Inferior herb drugs: Assistant herbs or poisons that are used mainly for treating diseases and cannot be taken for a long duration. They include Aconiti Radix, Rhei Rhizoma, and Persicae Semen.

In the Tang Dynasty (A.D. 618 to 905), Chinese therapies were affected by Indian medicine due to cultural exchange, and the number of drugs was increased. At that time, the government compiled the drug dictionary, *Hsin Hsiu Pen Tsao* (Revised Herbs, A.D. 659), which contained a collection of 850 varieties. In the Ming Dynasty (A.D. 1368 to 1628), the famous naturalist Li Shih Chen wrote *Pen Tsao Kang Mu* (Catalog of Medicinal Herbs, A.D. 1590) which contained an enlarged collection of 1,898 varieties. Presently, Chinese physicians employ about 520 varieties of herbs, among which about 200 are important.

Various herbs possess specific characteristics, which are called the "Four Properties and Five Flavors" in Chinese medicine. The Four Properties are the "chill" and "cool" of Yin and the "lukewarm" and "heat" of Yang, with an intermediate "level." Diseases with fever should be treated with the chill and cool herbs, while the chill and cool diseases should be treated with the herbs of heat. The Five Flavors are **Acrid, Sour, Sweet, Bitter, and Salty.** According to Chinese medicine, the acrid flavor is dispersing, the sour is astringent, the sweet is moderating, the bitter is strengthening, the salty is yielding, and the plain taste is moistening. The above herb characteristics have been accepted since ancient times even though scientific literature on their pharmacological interpretation is still lacking. Although many chemical constituents of Chinese herbs are known, each plant contains many more complex components, among which the one extracted is often not the most effective. Since each prescription of Chinese physicians contains four to twelve

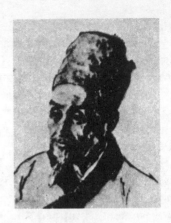

RIGHT—Li Shih-Chen, A.D. 1518-1953, China's greatest naturalist. He compiled the *Pen Ts'ao Kang Mu*, the General Catalog of Herbs, a work that took him forty years to complete.

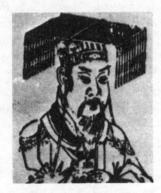

LEFT—Huang Ti, the "Yellow Emperor," the medical expert of 2674 B.C. From a wood carving.

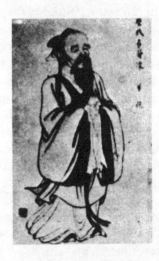

RIGHT—Hua To, A.D. 110-207, invented anaesthesia and developed anatomy in Chinese medicine and is therefore called "the father of surgery" in Chinese history. He used the anaesthetic property of coine and used Indian hemp in surgery.

herbs or more, the determination of its chemical reactions in the living body after combination and cooking of the herbs is a formidable challenge in research. In fact, the main reason Chinese medicine has not been able to enter the kingdom of science is the complexity of the scientific study necessary to explain the therapeutic mechanisms of herb formulas.

Chinese herbs and prescriptions, according to the findings of this author's experiments, have very low toxicity; generally, their LD50 is about 2 to 5 grams per kilogram of bodyweight. This is the reason Chinese medicine will exist far into the future. Modern drugs used by Western practitioners are effective, but when administered over a long period of time, will cause side effects and toxic states which can be harmful to the human body. Our Introduction of Chinese medicine has two main goals, instruction in the use of effective herbal formulas with minimum side effects and the joining of Chinese and Western medicines so that better therapeutic results and health may be available for all.

NOTICE

The therapies discussed in this book are strictly adjunctive or complementary to medical treatment. Self-treatment for a serious ailment can be dangerous. Therefore, you are urged to seek the advice of a Chinese herbal doctor or the best medical assistance available whenever it is needed.

HOW TO USE THIS BOOK

(Publisher's Foreword)

This book is basically a handbook of Chinese herbal medicine, which, unlike Western medicine, treats disease symptoms with mainly non-toxic drugs. A person can thereby treat himself without even knowing the name of his disease, and this handbook is ideal for such self-treatment.

1. Read the author's "Preface" and the "Brief Introduction to Chinese Medicine" for basic orientation to the Chinese approach.

2. Find your illness in Part I.

3. Choose the appropriate herbal formula.

4. Secure that formula from a Chinese drugstore or a health food store in your city - or through a chinese physician or herbal supplier such as the Brion Herb Corporation, 9250 Jeronimo Rd., Irvine, CA 92718, 1-800-333-HERB.

5. Take the appropriate formula.

This book is keyed to the products of the Sun Ten Pharmaceutical Works Co., Ltd., of Taiwan, the world's most important supplier of scientifically prepared Chinese herb formulas. The names of all formulas are given in both English and Chinese to avoid error.

Part II gives the exact composition, effects, and usages of each formula.

Parts III and IV give you botanical information on the herbs used in the Chinese formulas, including the chemical components. Your Western physician may find this of particular interest.

If you are a Westerner, "Diagnostic Outlines for the 13 Most Commonly Used Chinese Formulas" will introduce you to the very simple and practical manner by which Chinese medicine arrives at diagnoses.

Chinese herbal medicines are of low toxicity and have been used safely for thousands of years. Today it is estimated that approximately one billion persons in Southeast Asia regularly use Chinese herb formulas. Obviously, any possible risk in their usage must be so low as to be considered nonexistent, however, neither the author nor the publishers can assume any liability, express or implied, for your own self-treatment with the herbs and formulas discussed in this book. Consult your own physician as to your own specific situation.

In sum, treating yourself with Chinese herbal formulas is simple: you merely take the formula appropriate to your symptoms.

PART I

Differentiation of Illnesses and Chinese Herbal Formulas Appropriate For Their Treatment

RESPIRATORY DISORDERS

I. Common Cold

A. Mild

1. Ko-Ken-Tang   葛根湯 [101]
(Pueraria Combination)
Suitable for headache, fever, shivering without sweat, and aching in the shoulders.

2. Shih-Shen-Tang   十神湯 [10]
(M.H. and Cimicifuga Combination)
A modification of Ko-Ken-Tang, it is taken for fever, severe chill, headache, cough, gasping, and skin eruptions.

3. Ma-Huang-Tang   麻黃湯 [79]
(M.H. Combinations)
To be taken for influenza, high fever, headache, and arthralgia.

4. Sang-Chu-Yin   桑菊飲 [117]
(Morus and Chrysanthemum Combination)
Frequently used for subtropical "warm-wind disease" and tropical common cold.

1

B. Severe

1. Chai-Hu-Kuei-Chih-Tang　　　　柴胡桂枝湯
(Bupleurum and Cinnamon Combination)
Kuei-Chih-TangAndHsiao-Chai-Hu-Tang
This combined formula of **Kuei-Chih-Tang**
(Cinnamon Combination) and **Hsiao-Chai-Hu-Tang** (Minor Bupleurum Combination), to be taken for a lingering cold with mild fever.

2. Chai-Ko-Chiai-Chi-Tang　　　　柴葛解肌湯 ⁶¹
(Bupleurum and Pueraria Combination)
To be taken for headache, nasal dryness, thirst, pain in the hands and feet, and a large fast pulse.

C. In Those
of Delicate Constitution

1. Hsiang-Su-San　　　　　　香蘇散 ⁵³
(Cyperus and Perilla Formula)
To be taken for the common cold by those having gastrointestinal weakness.

2. Ma-Huang-Hsi-Hsin-Fu-Tzu-Tang 麻黃細辛附子湯 ⁸⁰
(M.H. and Asarum Combination)
It is frequently used by the elderly, the delicate, and those who are easily chilled.

D. With Cough

1. Hsiao-Ching-Lung-Tang　　　　小青龍湯 ¹⁸
(Blue Dragon Combination)
To be taken for persistent cough with large amounts of phlegm.

E. With Headache

1. Chuan-Chiung-Cha-Tiao-San   川芎茶調散 [13]
(Cnidium and Tea Formula)
This is commonly used for migraines, and vertigo due to the
common cold.

II. Bronchitis

A. Moist Cough

1. Hsiao-Ching-Lung-Tang   小青龍湯 [18]
(Minor Blue Dragon Combination)
To be taken for persistent cough, stridor, watery sputum,
congestion, headache, and chest pain.

2. Hsiao-Chai-Hu-Tang   小柴胡湯 [19]
(Minor Bupleurum Combination)
To be taken for mild fever, bitter taste, chest fullness, cough,
and sticky phlegm.

3. Ling-Kan-Chiang-Wei-Hsin-Hsia-Jen-Tang
(Hoelen and Schizandra   苓甘薑味辛夏仁湯 [55]
Combination)
To be taken for some chronic diseases of the elderly who have
a delicate constitution, frequent urination, chills, edema, and
anemia.

B. Harsh Cough

1. Mai-Men-Tung-Tang   麥門冬湯 [31]
(Ophiopogon Combination)
To be taken for a harsh cough without phlegm, but with dry
skin, and facial redness.

2. Pan-Hsia-Hou-Pu-Tang　　　　　　半夏厚朴湯 [30]
*(Pinellia and Magnolia
Combination)*
To be taken for moist and harsh cough with itching and pain
in the throat.

3. Ma-Hsing-Kan-Shih-Tang　　　　麻杏甘石湯 [77]
M.H. and Almond Combination)
This combination is taken at the onset of a hacking cough with
lingering sputum. It is especially effective for childhood
asthma.

4. Ching-Fei-Tang　　　　　　　　清肺湯 [85]
*(Platycodon and Fritillaria
Combination)*
To be taken for chronic hacking cough with lingering sputum.

III. Asthma

1. Ting-Chuan-San　　　　　　　　定喘散 [52]
(M.H. and Ginkgo Formula)
To be taken for wheezing, irritability, and loss of appetite.

2. Hua-Kai-San　　　　　　　　　華蓋散 [89]
(M.H. and Morus Combination)
To be taken for congestion and cough, chest fullness, stiffness
of the neck and back, and nasal congestion.

3. Shen-Mi-Tang　　　　　　　　神秘湯 [58]
M.H. and Magnolia Combination)
To be used over a long period for severe cough and difficulty
in breathing.

4. Ma-Huang-Hsi-Hsin-Fu-Tzu-Tang 麻黃細辛附子湯 [80]
(M.H. and Asarum Combination)
To be taken by those having a delicate constitution with severe
chills and headache.

4

IV. Tuberculosis and Pleurisy

1. Hsiao-Chai-Hu-Tang　　　　　　　小柴胡湯 19
(Minor Bupleurum Combination)
Chai-Hu-Kuei-Chih-Tang　　　　　柴胡桂枝湯 59
(Bupleurum and Cinnamon Combination)
Chai-Hsien-Tang　　　　　　　　　柴陷湯 115
*(Bupleurum and Scute
Combination)*
To be taken for early tuberculosis and pleurisy with mild fever
and loss of appetite.

2. Pu-Chung-I-Chi-Tang　　　　　　補中益氣湯 96
*(Ginseng and Astragalus
Combination)*
To be taken for tuberculosis and pleurisy with a tendency
towards fatigue, night sweats, and loss of appetite.

3. Mai-Men-Tung-Tang　　　　　　　麥門冬湯 81
(Ophiopogon Combination)
To be taken for sticky sputum and dry mouth. In cases with
hemoptysis, add Rehmannia, Gelatin, and Coptis.

4. Tzu-Yin-Chiang-Ho-Tang　　　　滋陰降火湯 121
(Phellodendron Combination)
To be taken for mild facial darkness, dry mouth, severe
cough, and spitting of blood.

5. Huang-Chi-San　　　　　　　　　黃解散 86
(Coptis and Scute Formula)
To be taken for sudden hemoptysis.

DIGESTIVE DISORDERS

I. Esophageal

1. Pan-Hsai-Hou-Pu-Tang　　　　半夏厚朴湯 [30]
*(Pinellia and Magnolia
Combination)*
To be taken for esophageal constriction and the sensation of
foreign matter in the throat.

2. Li-Ke-Tang　　　　利膈湯 [112]
*(Pinellia and Gardenia
Combination)*
To be taken for esophageal constriction and difficulty in
swallowing.

II. Gastrointestinal

1. Huang-Lien-Tang
(Coptis Combination)　　　　黃連湯
To be taken for a sensation of heavy pressure in the stomach,
sour stomach, nausea, loss of appetite, and white coating on
the tongue.

2. Ping-Wei-San　　　　　　　　平胃散 [37]
(Magnolia and Ginger Formula)
To be taken for gastric distension, nausea, vomiting, borborygmus after eating, temporary diarrhea, and indigestion.

3. Pan-Hsieh-Liu-Chun-Tzu-Tang　　　半瀉六君子湯 [33]
*(Pinellia and Ginseng six
Combination)*
To be taken for loss of appetite, tendency towards fatigue, and vomiting.

4. Shen-Chiang-Hsieh-Hsin-Tang　　　生薑瀉心湯 [34]
(Pinellia and Ginger Combination)
To be taken for hardness beneath the heart, stomach fullness, sighing, and sour stomach.

5. An-Chung-San　　　　　　　　安中散 [41]
(Cardamon and Fennel Formula)
This is taken by those of nervous constitution who have gastrointestinal discomfort and nausea.

6. Chai-Hu-Kuei-Chih-Tang　　　　柴胡桂枝湯 [59]
*(Bupleurum and Cinnamon
Combination)*
It is effective for aching beneath the heart, fever, distention and tenseness of the abdominal muscles.

7. Jen-Sheng-Tang
*(Ginseng and Ginger
Combination)*　　　　　　　　人參湯
To be taken for chilled extremities, pallor and gastrointestinal weakness.

7

8. Wu-Chu-Yu-Tang　　　　　　　　吳茱萸湯 [48]
(Evodia Combination)
To be taken for gastric weakness, frequent severe headaches, and vomiting.

III. Gastroptosis

1. Liu-Chun-Tzu-Tang　　　　　　六君子湯 [24]
(Major Six Herbs Combination)

Pan-Hsieh-Liu-Chun-Tzu-Tang　　半瀉六君子湯 [33]
(Pinellia and Ginseng
Six Combination)
To be taken for delicate constitution, loss of appetite, and stomach fullness after eating.

2. Pan-Hsia-Hou-Pu-Tang　　　　半夏厚朴湯 [30]
(Pinellia and Magnolia
Combination)
To be taken by women who have had several childbirths with resultant relaxation of the abdominal wall, stomach fullness, abdominal ache, a feeling of heaviness in the head, insomnia, and emotional instability.

3. Pu-Chung-I-Chi-Tang　　　　　補中益氣湯 [96]
(Ginseng and Astragalus
Combination)
This is good for gastrointestinal weakness and gastroptosis.

IV. Diarrhea

1. Kan-Tsao-Hsieh-Hsin-Tang　　　甘草瀉心湯 [39]
(Pinellia and Licorice
Combination)

8

Shen-Chiang-Hsieh-Hsin-Tang
(Pinellia and Ginger
Combination)　　　　　　　　生薑瀉心湯 [34]

Pan-Hsia-Hsieh-Hsin-Tang
(Pinellia Combination)　　　　半夏瀉心湯 [32]
All are effective for hardness beneath the heart, borborygmus,
diarrhea, nausea, vomiting, and occasional stomachache.

2. Liu-Chun-Tzu-Tang
(Major Six Herbs Combination)　六君子湯 [24]

Pan-Hsieh-Liu-Chun-Tzu-Tang
(Pinellia and Ginseng
Six Combination)　　　　　　　半瀉六君子湯
To be taken for frequent diarrhea, loss of appetite,
gastrointestinal fullness, and hiccoughs. If there is vomiting,
Pan-Hsieh-Liu-Chun-Tzu-Tang should be used.

3. Chen-Wu-Tang
(Vitality Combination)　　　　　眞武湯 [63]
To be taken by the elderly or those having anemia and chilling
of the hands and feet, stomachache, and diarrhea after meals.

4. Wu-Ling-San　　　　　　　　五苓散 [26]
(Hoelen Five Herbs Formula)
To be taken for thirst, stomach ache, vomiting, and watery
diarrhea in young children.

5. Ko-Ken-Huang-Lien-Huang-Chin-Tang
(Pueraria, Coptis and
Scute Combination)　　　　葛根黃連黃芩湯 [102]
To be taken for sunstroke, bacillary dysentery, stomachache,
and enteritis.

V. Habitual Constipation

1. Ta-Chai-Hu-Tang   大柴胡湯 [15]
(Major Bupleurum Combination)
To be taken by those having a strong constitution with good appetite, but frequent constipation and abdominal distention.

2. San-Huang-Hsieh-Hsin-Tang   三黃瀉心湯 [12]
(Coptis and Rhubarb Combination   （三黃錠）
To be taken for facial flushing, internal heat, nervousness, emotional instability, and constipation.

3. Ma-Tzu-Jen-Wan   麻子仁丸 [76]
(Almond and Cannabis Formula)
To be taken for habitual constipation of the elderly, or of the delicate with dry skin.

4. Hsiao-Chien-Chung-Tang   小建中湯 [20]
*(Minor Cinnamon and
Peony Combination)*
To be taken for constipation in young children.

5. Tang-Kuei-Shao-Yao-San   當歸芍藥散 [99]
*(Tang-Kuei and
Peony Formula)*
To be taken for constipation in pregnant women, which is often the cause of a difficult delivery.

6. Chia-Wei-Hsiao-Yao-San   加味逍遙散 [36]
*(Bupleurum and
Peony Formula)*
To be taken by women with menopausal symptoms and those with disorders of the autonomic nervous system.

VI. Vomiting

1. Hsiao-Pan-Hsia-Chia-Fu-Ling-Tang 小半夏加茯苓湯 [17]
*(Pinellia and Hoelen
Combination)*
It is effective for nausea and vomiting, especially when these
symptoms are present in pregnant women.

2. Wu-Ling-San 五苓散 [26]
(Hoelen Five Herbs Formula)
To be taken for acute "evil-wind" gastroenteritis of young
children, thirst, and decrease in urine.

VII. Stomach Cancer

1. Lo-Shih-Shu 樂適舒 [104]
(W.T.T.C.)
To be taken for early stomach cancer and for prevention of a
relapse. Its frequent use with Liu-Chun-Tzu-Tang (Major Six
Herbs Combination) may increase appetite.

VIII. Appendicitis

1. Chai-Hu-Kuei-Chih-Tang 柴胡桂枝湯 [59]
*(Bupleurum and Cinnamon
Combination)*
To be taken for early appendicitis with persistent ache in the
right lower abdomen.

2. Ta-Huang-Mu-Tan-Pi-Tang 大黃牡丹皮湯 [16]
(Rhubarb and Moutan Combination)
To be taken for swelling in the lower abdomen, and
constipation.

IX. Liver Disorders, Jaundice, and Gallstones

1. Ta-Chai-Hu-Tang　　　　　　　大柴胡湯 15
(Major Bupleurum Combination)
To be taken by those having an average constitution, but a tendency towards fatigue, pain in the liver when pressure is applied, and frequent constipation. It is also good for gallstones.

2. Hsiao-Chai-Hu-Tang　　　　　小柴胡湯 19
(Minor Bupleurum Combination)
It is effective for chest distension, a tendency towards fatigue, and loss of appetite.

3. Pu-Chung-I-Chi-Tang　　　　補中益氣湯 96
(Ginseng and Astragalus
Combination)
To be taken for a tendency towards anemia, severe fatigue, and loss of appetite. Frequent use will produce good results.

4. Chai-Hu-Kuei-Chih-Tang　　柴胡桂枝湯 59
(Bupleurum and Cinnamon
Combination)
To be taken for painful gallstones and cholecystitis. It should be used frequently, even after the pain has receded.

5. Chai-Hu-Kuei-Chih-Kan-Chiang-Tang
(Bupleurum' Cinnamon and　柴胡桂枝乾薑湯 61
Ginger Combination)
To be taken for fever, sleepiness, gasping due to weakness. It is especially effective for severe fatigue.

6. Yin-Chen-Hao-Tang　　　　　茵陳蒿湯 64
(Capillaris Combination)
To be taken for early jaundice, fever, and constipation.

12

7. Yin-Chen-Wu-Ling-San   茵陳五苓散 [65]
(Capillaris & Hoelen
Five Formula)
This combined formula of Yin-Chen-Hao-Tang (Capillaris Combination) and Wu-Ling-San 五苓散 , (Hoelen Five Herbs Formula), is used for thirst and difficult urination.

8. Chai-Ling-Tang   柴苓湯 [114]
(Bupleurum and Hoelen
Combination)
This combined formula of Hsiao-Chai-Hu-Tang (Minor Bupleurum Combination) and Wu-Ling-San (Hoelen Five Herbs Formula), is used for hepatomegaly, thirst, and difficult urination.

9. Shao-Yao-Kan-Tsao-Tang   芍藥甘草湯 [46]
(Peony and Licorice
Combination)
To be taken for recurrent gallstones.

10. Chia-Wei-Hsiao-Yao-San   加味逍遙散 [36]
(Bupleurum and Peony
Formula)
To be taken by those with a tendency towards fatigue, emotional instability, insomnia, and early cirrhosis without jaundice and abdominal ascites.

CIRCULATORY SYSTEM DISORDERS

I. Cardiac

1. Chai-Hu-Chia-Lung-Ku-Mu-Li-Tang
(Bupleurum and 柴胡加龍骨牡蠣湯 [62]
Dragon-Bone Combination)
To be taken for gasping respiration with severe insomnia, emotional instability, and nervousness.

2. Fang-Feng-Tung-Sheng-San
(Siler Formula) 防風通聖散 [44]
To be taken by those having an obese constitution and cardiac disorder and shortness of breath at any slight exertion.

3. Ling-Kuei-Chu-Kan-Tang
(Atractylodes and Hoelen 苓桂朮甘湯 [54]
Combination)
It is effective for vertigo, dizziness on standing, and shortness of breath.

4. Mu-Fang-Chi-Tang
(Stephania and Ginseng 木防己湯 [21]
Combination)
To be taken for difficulty in breathing, stridor, edema, hardness beneath the heart, endocarditis, and vascular disease.

5. Chiu-Kan-Tsao-Tang   炙甘草湯 [51]
(Licorice Combination)
To be taken for palpitation, gasping respiration, stagnant pulse, thirst, limbs fever, anemia, and dry skin.

6. Pien-Chih-Hsin-Chi-Yin   變製心氣飲 [110]
*(Areca and Evodia
Combination)*
To be taken for difficult urination, edema, palpitation, shortness of respiration, heaviness of head, distension. After taking

Mu-Fang-Chi-Tang   木防己湯 [21]
*(Stephania and Ginseng
Combination)*
without results, this formula should be used.

II. Hypertension and Arteriosclerosis

There is no hypotensive in Chinese formulas. Although the primary aim of Western Medicine is to decrease blood pressure, Chinese formulas first adjust the imbalance within the whole body; the blood pressure becomes normal when there is a balance in the body.

1. Ta-Chai-Hu-Tang   大柴胡湯 [15]
(Major Bupleurum Combination)
To be taken by those having a strong constitution with symptoms of chest distention, pressure in the chest, constipation, and shoulder stiffness.

2. San-Huang-Hsieh-Hsin-Tang
(Coptis and Rhubarb Combination)

三黃瀉心湯 [12]

To be taken for severe facial flushing, internal heat with emotional instability, congestion, insomnia, nervousness, and a tendency towards constipation. In cases without constipation, the patient should use

Huang-Lien-Chiai-Tu-Tang
(Coptis and Scute Combination).

黃連解毒湯 [86]

3. Chai-Hu-Chia-Lung-Ku-Mu-Li-Tang
(Bupleurum and Dragon-Bone Combination)

柴胡加龍骨牡蠣湯 [69]

This is effective for palpitations, vertigo, and nervousness resulting in wheezing.

4. Pa-Wei-Ti-Huang-Wan
(Rehmannia Eight Formula)

八味地黃丸 [7]

It is effective for hypertension in the elderly with thirst, fatigue, and frequent urination at night.

5. Ling-Kuei-Chu-Kan-Tang
(Atractylodes and Hoelen Combination)

苓桂朮甘湯 [54]

This is effective for vertigo or severe wheezing with headache.

6. Kou-Teng-San
(Gambir Formula)

鈎藤散 [93]

To be taken for morning headache, tinnitus due to frequent migraine, chest distension, amnesia, and especially cerebral arteriosclerosis.

7. Chi-Wu-Chiang-Hsia-Tang 七物降下湯 [5]
(Tang-Kuei and Gambir Combination)
To be taken by the patient of a delicate constitution with arteriolas nephrosclerosis, albuminuria, shortness of breath, and headache.

8. Fang-Feng-Tung-Sheng-San 防風通聖散 [44]
(Siler Formula)
To be taken by those of obese constitution with shoulder stiffness, headache, and a tendency towards constipation. It is also a hypertension preventive.

9. Hsu-Ming-Tang 續命湯 [109]
(M.H. and Ginseng Combination)
To be taken for apraxia and aphasia, sensory disorder, and hemiplegia due to a stroke.

III. Hypotension

1. Pu-Chung-I-Chi-Tang 補中益氣湯 [96]
(Ginseng and Astragalus Combination)
To be taken by those with a tendency towards anemia, fatigue, and loss of appetite. It is a famous tonic formula for nourishing the body and the blood.

2. Tang-Kuei-Shao-Yao-San 當歸芍藥散 [99]
(Tang-Kuei and Peony Formula)
To be taken by those with a tendency towards chills, anemia, and pallor. It is a blood tonic, and it increases blood pressure.

3. Ling-Kuei-Chu-Kan-Tang
*(Atractylodes and
Hoelen Combination)*

苓桂朮甘湯 [54]

To be taken for vertigo, asthenopia, or wheezing. For those having anemia and chills, it is administered in combination with

Tang-Kuei-Shao-Yao-San
*(Tang-Kuei and
Peony Formula)*

當歸芍藥散 [99]

4. Chen-Wu-Tang
(Vitality Combination)

眞武湯 [63]

To be taken by the patient with a tendency towards fatigue, diarrhea, chilling of the limbs, vertigo, and weakness.

5. Pan-Hsia-Pai-Chu-Tien-Ma-Tang
*(Pinellia and Gastrodia
Combination)*

半夏白朮天麻湯 [31]

To be taken by the patient having gastroptosis or gastrointestinal weakness, with a tendency towards fatigue, chilling of the limbs, vertigo, headache, nausea, and sleepiness after eating.

UROLOGICAL DISORDERS

I. Kidney and Bladder

1. Wu-Ling-San　　　　　　　　　　　五苓散 [26]
(Hoelen Five Herbs Formula)
To be taken for acute and chronic kidney conditions; but for
the chronic cases, its combination with

Hsiao-Chai-Hu-Tang　　　　　　　　小柴胡湯 [19]
(Minor Bupleurum Combination)
may produce better results. It is effective for the primary
stages of acute nephritis, thirst, and difficulty in urination.

2. Chu-Ling-Tang　　　　　　　　　　豬苓湯 [88]
(Polyporus Combination)
To be taken regularly for cystitis, urethritis, difficulty in
defecation, albuminuria, hematuria, and painful urination.

3. Tang-Kuei-Shao-Yao-San　　　　當歸芍藥散 [99]
*(Tang-Kuei and
Peony Formula)*
It is very effective for edema in pregnancy, and for
albuminuria. It is also effective for a tendency towards anemia
with albuminuria and edema.

4. Pa-Wei-Ti-Huang-Wan
(Rehmannia Eight Formula)

八味地黃丸 [7]

To be taken for kidney atrophy or senile nephritis. It is also effective for edema, tinnitus, hypertension, difficulty in urination, thirst, pain near the waist, fatigue, diabetes, and prostatomegaly.

5. Hsiao-Chai-Hu-Tang
(Minor Bupleurum Combination)

小柴胡湯 [19]

To be taken by those with chronic nephritis. It is frequently taken with

Wu-Ling-San
(Hoelen Five Herb Formula)
or

五苓散 [26]

Chu-Ling-Tang
(Polyporus Combination).

豬苓湯 [88]

6. Fen-Hsiao-Tang
(Hoelen and Alisma Combination)

分消湯 [22]

To be taken for fluid stagnancy in the abdomen, hardness and tenseness in the abdomen, and a sunken-strong pulse.

7. Lung-Tan-Hsieh-Kan-Tang
(Gentiana Combination)

龍膽瀉肝湯 [105]

To be taken for cystitis, inflammation and suppuration in the lower abdomen and genital areas, difficulty in urination, turbid urine, and leucorrhea.

ENDOCRINE AND BLOOD DISORDERS

I. Diabetes

1. Liu-Wei-Ti-Huang-Wan
(Rehmannia Six Formula)

六味地黃丸 [23]

To be taken for vertigo, tinnitus, spermatorrhea, weakness at the waist and knees, thirst, and diabetes.

2. Pa-Wei-Ti-Huang-Wan
(Rehmannia Eight Formula)

八味地黃丸 [7]

To be taken by those of delicate constitution with dimness of vision, thirst, dry skin, impotence, lumbago, and tinnitus. It is suitable for senile diabetes.

3. Pai-Hu-Chia-Jen-Shen-Tang
(Ginseng and Gypsum Combination)

白虎加人參湯 [29]

To be taken for severe thirst, frequent urination, tendency towards fatigue, and loss of weight.

4. Szu-Chun-Tzu-Tang
(Major Four Herbs Combination)

四君子湯 [27]

To be taken for weakness, loss of appetite, anemia, and edema in the lower limbs.

5. Fang-Feng-Tung-Sheng-San
(Siler and Platycodon Formula)　　　　防風通聖散 [44]

To be taken by those of obese and strong constitution as a diabetes preventive.

II. Obesity

1. Fang-Feng-Tung-Sheng-San
(Siler and Platycodon Formula)　　　　防風通聖散 [44]

To be taken for those of obese constitution with constipation. It is also effective for those whose obesity is related to overconsumption of meat.

2. Fang-Chi-Huang-Chi-Tang
(Stephania and Astragalus　　　　防己黃耆湯 [43]
Combination)

To be taken by those of obese constitution with flaccid muscles, tendencies towards fatigue and prespiration, heart weakness, and edema. The majority of the patients are women.

III. Anemia

1. Szu-Wu-Tang
(Tang-Kuei Four　　　　四物湯
Combination)

This is a tonic for nourishing the body and the blood.

2. Szu-Chun-Tzu-Tang
(Major Four Herbs　　　　四君子湯 [7]
Combination)

To be taken by those of delicate constitution for anemia and a tendency towards fatigue.

3. Shih-Chuan-Ta-Pu-Tang
(Ginseng and Tang-Kuei Ten Combination)

十全大補湯 '

This is a combined formula of Pa-Chen-Tang (Tang-Kuei and Ginseng Eight Combination) with Cinnamomi Ramulus and Astragali Radix. It is taken for weakness, anemia, and dryness of the mouth.

4. Tang-Kuei-Shao-Yao-San
(Tang-Kuei and Peony Formula)

當歸芍藥散 [99]

To be taken by those of delicate constitution with anemia, and it is especially effective for pregnant women.

5. Jen-Shen-Tang
(Ginseng and Ginger Combination)

人參湯 [2]

To be taken by those with anemia, loss of appetite, and a tendency towards diarrhea.

6. Kuei-Pi-Tang
(Ginseng and Longan Combination)

歸脾湯 [107]

To be taken for chronic anemia, insomnia, amnesia, palpitations, and asthenia due to hemorrhage.

IV. Ephidrosis

1. Wu-Ling-San
(Hoelen Five Herbs Formula)

五苓散 [26]

To be taken for thirst, ephidrosis, and difficulty in urination.

2. Fang-Chi-Huang-Chi-Tang
(Stephania and Astragalus Combination)

防己黃耆湯

To be taken by those of obese constitution who have a tendency towards fatigue and ephidrosis. The majority of patients are female.

3. Kuei-Chih-Chia-Huang-Chi-Tang   桂枝加黃耆湯 [71]
(Cinnamon and Astragalus Combination)

To be taken by those of delicate constitution who are susceptible to colds and ephidrosis.

V. Hyperthyroidism

1. Chih-Kan-Tsao-Tang   炙甘草湯 [51]
(Licorice Combination)

To be taken for occasional palpitation and obstructed pulse.

2. Chai-Hu-Chia-Lung-Ku-Mu-Li-Tang   [62]
(Bupleurum and   柴胡加龍骨牡蠣湯
Dragon-Bone Combination)

To be taken for chest distension, abdominal distension, excitability, fatigue palpitations, and insomnia during the initial stage of an illness.

VI. Beriberi

1. Yueh-Pi-Chia-Chu-Tang   越婢加朮湯 [92]
(Atractylodes Combination)

To be taken for edema of the lower limbs, perspiration, thirst and difficulty in urination.

2. Chiu-Ping-Wu-Fu-Tang   九檳吳茯湯 [8]
(Areca Combination)

To be taken for fatigue, tired feet, rapid respirations, and edema.

JOINT AND NERVE DISORDERS

I. Neuralgia and Arthritis (Rheumatism)

1. Ko-Ken-Tang　　　　　　　　　葛根湯 [101]
(Pueraria Combination)
It is effective for primary neuralgia, rheumatism, aching shoulders, and facial neuralgia.

2. Ma-Hsing-I-Kan-Tang　　　　　麻杏薏甘湯 [78]
(M.H. and Coix Combination)
It is effective for arthritis, for muscle aches, and especially for chronic rheumatism.

3. I-Yi-Jen-Tang　　　　　　　　薏苡仁湯 [106]
(Coix Combination)
To be taken for febrile swelling.

4. Kuei-Chih-Chia-Chu-Fu-Tang　桂枝加朮附湯 [68]
(Cinnamon and
Aconite Combination)
It is effective for neuralgia and rheumatism of the chill phobia constitution (fear of becoming chilled), especially when there is aching of the part or difficult movement of the limbs.

5. Kuei-Chih-Shao-Yao-Chih-Mu-Tang
(Cinnamon and
Anemarrhena Combination)　　桂枝芍藥知母湯

To be taken for chronic arthrophyma, atrophy of the surrounding muscle, and dry skin.

6. Pa-Wei-Ti-Huang-Wan
(Rehmannia Eight Formula)　　八味地黃丸 [7]

It is effective for thirst, tendency towards fatigue, and aching and numbness near the waist and in the feet.

7. Tao-Ho-Chen-Chi-Tang
(Persica and Rhubarb
Combination)　　桃核承氣湯 [72]

It is effective for those having sciatic neuralgia accompanied by dark red face, headache, constipation, and menstrual disorder.

8. Shu-Ching-Huo-Hsieh-Tang
(Clematis and Stephania
Combination)　　疏經活血湯 [91]

To be taken for chronic sciatic neuralgia and arthroneuralgia, especially below the waist.

9. Shu-Ching-Li-An-San
(Clematis and Carthamus
Formula)　　舒筋立安散 [90]

To be taken for chronic arthroneuralgia, pain in the arms and legs, and neuralgia.

10. Tu-Huo-Chi-Sheng-Tang
(Tu-huo and Viscum
Combination)　　獨活寄生湯 [127]

To be taken for pain near the waist and in the knees, chills and weakness, difficulty in walking, and neuralgia.

26

II. Neurasthenia and Insomnia

Chai-Hu-Chia-Lung-Ku-Mu-Li-Tang
(Bupleurum and   柴胡加龍骨牡蠣湯 [62]
Dragon-Bone Combination)
To be taken for nervousness, emotional instability, insomnia, anxiety, palpitations, chest distension, and congestion.

2. Suan-Tsao-Jen-Tang   酸棗仁湯 [103]
(Zizyphus Combination)
To be taken to increase brain function and to relieve fatigue, stress, and insomnia.

3. Kuei-Pi-Tang   歸脾湯 [107]
(Ginseng and Longan
Combination)
To be taken for insomnia, amnesia, emotional instability, nervousness, fearfulness, palpitation, gastrointestinal weakness, and anemia.

4. I-Kan-San   抑肝散 [45]
(Bupleurum Formula)
To be taken by nervous and easily excitable patients with insomnia, mental instability, muscular spasm, and shivering.

5. Kan-Mai-Ta-Tsao-Tang   甘麥大棗湯 [38]
(Licorice and
Jujube Combination)
To be taken for hysteria in women with a tendency towards crying, coma, and manic behavior.

6. Tien-Wang-Pu-Hsin-Tang
(Ginseng and Zizyphus   天王補心丹 [25]
Formula)
To be taken to nourish the blood, to relieve anxiety due to stress, and for ephidrosis, emotional instability, constipation, amnesia, and nervous exhaustion in young people.

7. Wen-Tan-Tang
溫膽湯 [122]
Bamboo and Hoelen
Combination)

To be taken for insomnia, palpitation, anxiety, nervous exhaustion, and neurosis.

III. Vertigo

1. Ling-Kuei-Chu-Kan-Tang
苓桂朮甘湯 [54]
(Atractylodes and
Hoelen Combination)

To be taken for vertigo, headache, tinnitus, sea-sickness, and car-sickness. The addition of Gastrodia to this formula can produce better results.

2. Tang-Kuei-Shao-Yao-San
當歸芍藥散 [99]
(Tang-Kuei and Peony
Formula)

To be taken frequently for a feeling of heaviness in the head, anemia, and vertigo after childbirth.

3. Pan-Hsia-Pai-Chu-Tien-Ma-Tang 半夏白朮天麻湯 [31]
(Pinellia and Gastrodia
Combination)

To be taken by those of weak confirmation with chilling of the limbs, headache, and vertigo.

GYNECOLOGICAL DISORDERS

I. General

1. Tang-Kuei-Shao-Yao-San 　　當歸芍藥散 [99]
(Tang-Kuei and Peony Formula)

It is effective for aching shoulders, vertigo, polyuria, rough skin, and menstrual aberration in those of the chill confirmation.

2. Kuei-Chih-Fu-Ling-Wan 　　桂枝茯苓丸 [66]
(Cinnamon and Hoelen Formula)

It is effective for headache, vertigo, tinnitus, chills in the lower limbs, congestion, and menstrual irregularities in young women.

3. Pan-Hsia-Hou-Pu-Tang 　　半夏厚朴湯 [30]
(Pinellia and Magnolia Combination)

To be taken by neurasthenic women with a sensation of something being stuck in the throat or chest, nausea, and nervousness.

29

4. Tao-Ho-Chen-Chi-Tang
(Persica and Rhubarb Combination)

桃核承氣湯 [72]

To be taken by those of strong constitution with facial flushing and darkening, headache, vertigo, chilling in the lower abdomen, ache near the waist, constipation, and menstrual disorders.

5. Chia-Wei-Hsiao-Yao-San
(Bupleurum and Peony Formula)

加味逍遙散 [36]

To be taken for fatigue, tiredness of the limbs, chills, vertigo, insomnia, congestion, facial flushing, thirst, chilling of the back, and hot flushes. It is also effective for menopausal disorders.

6. Chiung-Kuei-Chiao-Ai-Tang
Tang-Kuei and Gelatin Combination)

芎歸膠艾湯 [47]

To be taken for anemia and by those of delicate constitution with uterine or hemorrhoidal bleeding.

II. Pregnancy and Childbirth

1. Hsiao-Pan-Hsia-Chia-Fu-Ling-Tang
(Pinellia and Hoelen Combination)

小半夏加茯苓湯 [17]

To be taken for early toxemia of pregnancy.

2. An-Tai-Yin
(Tang-Kuei and Parsley Combination)

（安胎飲） [57]

To be taken for vomiting during pregnancy, a feeling of heaviness in the head, vertigo, and premature contractions. It may be replaced by

Tang-Kuei-Shao-Yao-San
*(Tang-Kuei and
Peony Formula)*

當歸芍藥散 99

3. Shen-Hua-Tang
*(Tang-Kuei and Ginger
Combination)*
To be taken for nourishing the blood and for abdominal pain
after childbirth.

生化湯 35

4. Pu-Kung-Ying-Tang
(Dandelion Combination)
This formula is a lactagogue.

蒲公英湯 125

5. Shih-Wei-Pai-Tu-San
*(Bupleurum and Schizonepeta
Formula)*
To be taken for mastitis, with fever, pain in the breast,
swelling and suppuration. At the outset, the patient may take

十味敗毒散 11

Hsiao-Chai-Hu-Tang
(Minor Bupleurum Combination)
with Platycodon and Gypsum.

小柴胡湯 19

III. Infertility and Chill

1. Wen-Ching-Tang
*(Tang-Kuei and Evodia
Combination)*
To be taken for infertility, lack of vitality, chills, feverish
palms, dry lips, chilling near the waist, menstrual disorders,
leucorrhea, uterine bleeding, and menopausal disorders.

溫經湯 94

2. Tang-Kuei-Shao-Yao-San
*(Tang-Kuei and
Peony Formula)*

當歸芍藥散 [99]

To be taken by the women of delicate constitution with chills near the waist and in the feet, and an underdeveloped uterus and ovaries, and habitual abortion.

**3. Tang-Kuei-Szu-Ni-Chia-Wu-
Nhu-Yu-Shen-Chiang-Tang**
*(Tang-Kuei, Evodia and
Ginger Combination)*

當歸四逆加吳茱萸生薑湯

To be taken for chills near the waist and in the lower abdomen, abdominal distention, and frequent chilblain.

4. Jen-Sheng-Tang
*(Ginseng and Ginger
Combination)*

人參湯 [2]

To be taken by patients of both sexes having a delicate constitution and who often work in air-conditioned rooms. It is also effective for recurrent diarrhea.

IV. Endometritis

1. Lung-Tan-Hsieh-Kan-Tang
Gentiana Combination)

龍膽瀉肝湯 [105]

To be taken for suppurative endometritis, leucorrhea, turbid urine, difficulty in urination, and the tense abdomen.

2. Pa-Wei-Tai-Hsia-Fang
*(Tang-Kuei and Eight
Herbs Formula)*

八味帶下方 [6]

To be taken by the women of delicate constitution with chronic leucorrhea and anemia.

PEDIATRIC DISORDERS

I. Improving General Vitality

1. Hsiao-Chien-Chung-Tang
小建中湯 [20]
(Minor Cinnamon and Peony Combination)
This formula is good for children of delicate constitution. To be taken for bed-wetting, night crying, stomachache, and hernia. It is also effective for childhood constipation and diarrhea.

2. Hsiao-Chai-Hu-Tang
小柴胡湯 [19]
(Minor Bupleurum Combination)
To be taken for recurrent fever in infants, tonsillitis, bronchitis, otitis media, and inflammation of the throat.

3. Chai-Hu-Kuei-Chih-Tang
柴胡桂枝湯 [191]
(Bupleurum and Cinnamon Combination)
This is a combined formula of Hsiao-Chai-Hu-Tang (Minor Bupleurum Combination) and Kuei-Chih-Tang (Cinnamon Combination). To be taken for susceptibility to the common cold, nasal congestion, and rhinorrhea.

4. Liu-Chun-Tzu-Tang　　　　　　　六君子湯 [24]
*(Major Six Herbs
Combination)*
To be taken for gastrointestinal weakness, loss of appetite,
pallor, and lack of vigor.

II. Whooping Cough and Pediatric Asthma

1. Hsiao-Ching-Lung-Tang　　　　　小青龍湯 [18]
(Minor Blue Dragon Combination)
To be taken for a common cold, cough, rhinorrhea, sneezing,
and conjuctival congestion.

2. Ma-Hsig-Kan-Shih-Tang　　　　麻杏甘石湯 [77]
(M.H. and Almond Combination)
To be taken for severe cough, perspiration on the forehead,
thirst, and asthma in children.

3. Hsiao-Chai-Hu-Tang with [19]
Pan-Hsia-Hou-Pu-Tang　　小柴胡湯合半夏厚朴湯 [30]
*(Minor Bupleurum Combination plus Pinellia and Magnolia
Combination)*
To be taken for nervousness in children, lingering cough, and
emotional instability.

III. Indigestion

1. Wu-Ling-San　　　　　　　　　五苓散 [26]
(Hoelen Five Herbs Formula)
To be taken at the onset of indigestion for thirst, vomiting,
diarrhea, loss of appetite, and difficulty in urination.

2. Sheng-Ling-Pai-Chu-San　　　參苓白术散 [82]
*(Ginseng and Atractylodes
Formula)*
To be taken for gastrointestinal weakness, indigestion,
vomiting, or diarrhea.

IV. Night Crying

1. Kan-Mai-Ta-Tsao-Tang　　　　　甘麥大棗湯 [38]
*(Licorice and Jujube
Combination)*
To be taken for nervousness in infants, excitability, and night
crying.

V. Bed-wetting

1. Hsiao-Chien-Chung-Tang　　　　小建中湯 [20]
*(Minor Cinnamon and
Peony Combination)*
To be taken for abdominal weakness, thirst, difficulty in
urination, and bed-wetting.

SKIN DISORDERS

I. Urticaria

1. Ko-Ken-Tang   葛根湯 [101]
(Pueraria Combination)
To be taken at the onset of urticaria for inflammation, itching, and fever if present. In case there is constipation, add Rhubarb.

2. Hsiao-Ching-Lung-Tang   小青龍湯 [18]
(Minor Blue Dragon Combination)
To be taken for rhinorrhea, sneezing, and allergic rhinitis.

3. Hsiao-Chai-Hu-Tang   小柴胡湯 [19]
(Minor Bupleurum Combination)
To be taken for improving on obese constitution and for chest distension, with a feeling of tenseness beneath the heart.

4. Shih-Wei-Pai-Tu-San   十味敗毒散 [11]
(Bupleurum and Schizonepeta Formula)

Chin-Fang-Pai-Tu-San   荊防敗毒散 [74]
(Schizonepeta and Siler Formula)
Both of the above are effective for frequent urticaria.

5. Teng-Hua-Pai-Tu-San   燈花敗毒散 [126]
(Ludwigia Formula)
To be taken as a detoxifier, antiphlogistic, and diuretic. This is also used for primary urticaria.

6. Jen-Sheng-Pai-Tu-San   人參敗毒散 [4]
(Ginseng and Mentha
Formula)
To be taken by those having skin disease who are of delicate constitution.

II. Eczema

1. Wen-Ching-Yin   溫清飲 [95]
(Tang-Kuei and
Gardenia Combination)
To be taken for dry eczema, fever, and itching. This is a combined formula of:

Szu-Wu-Tang   四物湯 [28]
(Tang-Kuei Four Combination)
and

Huang-Lien-Chiai-Tu-Tang   黃連解毒湯 [86]
(Coptis and Scute Combination),
effective for stagnant blood and inflammation.

2. Hsiao-Feng-San   消風散 [75]
(Tang-Kuei and
Arctium Formula)
To be taken for chronic and recalcitrant eczema, moist eczema, inflammation, pruritis, and scabies.

3. Shih-Wei-Pai-Tu-San   十味敗毒散 [11]
(Bupleurum and Schizonepeta
Formula)
To be taken for chronic eczema.

III. Cosmetic (Facial) Uses

1. Tang-Kuei-Shao-Yao-San   當歸芎藥散 [99]
(Tang-Kuei and
Peony Formula)
To be taken by women with freckles around the eyes and nose, delicate constitution, pallor, and a tendency towards fatigue. Coix is often added to produce better results.

2. Kuei-Chich-Fu-Ling-Wan   桂枝茯苓丸 [66]
(Cinnamon and
Hoelen Formula)
To be taken by women of average constitution with endometritis or ovaritis.

3. Chia-Wei-Hsiao-Yao-San   加味逍遙散 [36]
(Bupleurum and Peony Formula)
To be taken after middle age by women with nervousness, emotional instability, a feeling of tiredness in the limbs, and chills with a feverish sensation.

4. Ching-Shang-Fang-Feng-Tang   清上防風湯 [84]
(Siler Combination)
To be taken by young people with acne, facial redness, and conjunctival congestion. Addition of 1.0 g. of Coix to this formula each time may produce better results.

GERIATRIC DISORDERS

1. Liu-Wei-Ti-Huang-Wan
(Rehmannia Six Formula)
Pa-Wei-Ti-Huang-Wan *(Rehmannia Eight Formula)*

六味地黃丸 ₂₃
八味地黃丸

To be taken for impotence, a tendency towards fatigue, chills near the waist, lumbago, sperma torrhea, thirst, and decreased sexual desire. It is effective for the elderly with prostatomegaly, nephrosclerosis, diabetes, lumbago, neuralgia, and cataract. Generally Liu-Wei-Ti-Huang-Wan is used. For the patient of delicate constitution, Pa-Wei-Ti-Huang-Wan is used.

2. Jen-Sheng-Yang-Yung-Tang
(Ginseng Nutritive Combination)
Shih-Chuan-Ta-Pu-Tang with Lu-Rong
(Ginseng and Tang-Kuei Combination with Cervus)

人參養榮湯 ₂
十全大補湯
加鹿茸

To be taken for rehabilitation of the elderly with a delicate constitution, amnesia, loss of appetite, fatigue, and loss of hair. Shih-Chuan-Ta-Pu-Tang with Lu-Rong is the more effective of the two.

3. Kuei-Chih-Chia-Lung-Ku-Mu-Li-Tang
(Cinnamon and
Dragon-Bone Combination)

桂枝加龍骨牡蠣湯

Chai-Hu-Chia-Lung-Ku-Mu-Li-Tang 62
(Bupleurum and 柴胡加龍骨牡蠣湯
Dragon-Bone Combination)
For those of average constitution, a tendency towards fatigue, excitability, congestion, palpitation, and frequent urination, the patient should take this formula or

Kuei-Chih-Chia-Lung-Ku-Mu-Li-Tang 69
(Cinnamon and 桂枝加龍骨牡蠣湯
Dragon-Bone Combination).
To be taken in cases involving chest distension and palpitation above the umbilicus.

4. Huan-Shao-Tan 還少丹 128
(Lycium Formula)
To be taken to increase vigor.

5. Chin-Sou-Ku-Ching-Wan 金鎖固精丸 50
(Lotus Stamen Formula)
To be taken for impotence, spermatorrhea, ache near the waist, tinnitus, and weakness of the limbs.

EYE DISORDERS

I. Conjunctivitis and Sty

1. Ko-Ken-Tang　　　　　　　　　葛根湯 [101]
(Pueraria Combination)
To be taken at the onset of inflammation, swelling, and pain
in the eye. In cases with constipation, add Chung-Huang-San
(Cnidium and Rhubarb Formula).

2. Yueh-Pi-Chia-Chu-Tang　　　　越婢加朮湯 [92]
(Atractylodes Combination)
To be taken for blepharitis with swelling, congestion, pain,
secretion, and lacrimation.

3. Hsiao-Ching-Lung-Tang　　　　小青龍湯 [18]
(Minor Blue Dragon Combination)
To be taken for conjuctivitis, congestion, and lacrimation.

4. Hsi-Kan-Ming-Mu-San　　　　洗肝明目湯 [56]
(Gardenia and Vitex Formula)
It is effective for keratitis.

II. Cataract

1. Pa-Wei-Ti-Huang-Wan　　　　八味地黄丸 [7]
(Rehmannia Eight Formula)
It is effective for cataract, ache and chills near the waist, and
especially for weakness of the limbs.

2. Tzu-Sheng-Ming-Mu-Tang　　　　滋腎明目湯 [97]
(Chrysanthemum Combination)
To be taken for impotence, weakness, eye disorders, asthenopia, and astigmatism.

III. Pseudo-Nearsightedness

1. Ling-Kuei-Chu-Kan-Tang　　　　苓桂朮甘湯 [54]
(Atractylodes and
Hoelen Combination)
To be taken for vertigo when standing. Those with thirst and difficulty in urination, should use

Wu-Ling-San　　　　　　　　　五苓散 [26]
(Hoelen Five Herbs Formula).

IV. Asthenopia

1. Hsiao-Chai-Hu-Tang　　小柴胡湯合苓桂朮甘湯 [54]
with Ling-Kuei-Chu-Kan-Tang
(Minor Bupleurum Combination
When used concurrently,
the two formulas are
effective against asthenopia.

EAR, NOSE, AND THROAT
DISORDERS

I. Nasal Suppuration and Chronic Rhinitis

1. Ching-Pi-Tang　　　　　　　　清鼻湯 [83]
(Pueraria Nasal Combination)
This is a good oral formula effective for nasal suppuration,
chronic rhinitis, and nasal congestion. To be taken by those
with a feeling of heaviness in the head, emotional instability,
and occasional suppuration.

2. Ko-Ken-Tang with Hsin-I　　葛根湯加辛夷、川芎 [123]
and Chuan-Chiung
(Pueraria and Magnolia Combination)
It is effective for nasal congestion and allergic rhinitis.

3. Ling-Kuei-Chu-Kan-Tang　　　苓桂朮甘湯 [54]
(Atractylodes and Hoelen
Combination)
To be taken by those with gastrointestinal weakness, a feeling
of heaviness in the head, vertigo, and tinnitus with nasal
suppuration. It may be taken with

Ko-Ken-Tang with　　　　葛根湯加辛夷、川芎 [121]
Hsin-I and Chuan-Chiung
(Pueraria and Magnolia Combination)

4. Shih-Wei-Pai-Tu-San   十味敗毒散 11
(Bupleurum and
Schizonepeta Formula)

Chin-Chiai-Lien-Chiao-Tang 荊芥連翹湯 73
(Schizonepeta and Forsythia
Combination)
Both of the above are effective for malodorous suppuration
having a tendency towards becoming chronic.

5. Hsin-I-Ching-Fei-Tang   辛夷清肺湯 49
(Magnolia and Gypsum
Combination)
Hsin-I-San   辛夷散 113
(Magnolia Formula)

Tsang-Erh-San   蒼耳散 124
(Xanthium Formula)
All are effective for nasal neoplasm, and nasal congestion.
When fever and aches are present, take:

Hsin-I-Ching-Fei-Tang   辛夷清肺湯 49
(Magnolia Gypsum Combination).

II. Otitis Media

1. Ko-Ken-Tang   葛根湯 101
(Pueraria Combination)
To be taken for acute otitis media with fever, and severe chills.

2. Hsiao-Chai-Hu-Tang 小柴胡湯 19
(Minor Bupleurum Combination)
To be taken for chronic otitis media, when there is bitter taste
in the mouth, white coating on the tongue, ear-ache, and
difficulty in hearing.

3. Huang-Chi-Chien-Chung-Tang　　黃耆建中湯 [87]
(Astragalus Combination)
To be taken for otitis media in infants, with continuous suppuration.

4. Tuo-Li-Hsiao-Tu-Yin　　托裏消毒飲 [42]
(Gleditschia Combination)
To be taken for chronic otitis media with continuous suppuration, weakness, and fatigue.

III. Tinnitus

1. Ling-Kuei-Chu-Kan-Tang　　苓桂朮甘湯 [54]
*(Atractylodes and Hoelen
Combination)*
To be taken by the patients with a feeling of heaviness in the head, vertigo, nervousness, and a tendency towards palpitation.

2. Tang-Kuei-Shao-Yao-San　　當歸芍藥散 [99]
*(Tang-Kuei and
Peony Formula)*
To be taken by women of delicate constitution who have chills and tinnitus.

3. Ta-Chai-Hu-Tang　　大柴胡湯 [15]
(Major Bupleurum Combination)

Fang-Feng-Tung-Sheng-San　　防風通聖散 [44]
*(Siler and Platycodon
Formula)*
Both of the above are effective for tinnitus due to arteriosclerosis and hypertension, a feeling of heaviness in the head, chest distension and constipation.

4. Tzu-Sheng-Tung-Erh-Tang　　　　滋腎通耳湯
(Scute Combination)

To be taken for tinnitus due to kidney disorder, and for difficulty in hearing.

IV. Tonsillitis

1. Ko-Ken-Tang　　　　　　　　葛根湯 [101]
(Pueraria Combination)

To be taken for sore throat with fever.

2. Ching-Liang-Yin　　　　　　　清涼飲 [118]
*(Gardenia and Mentha
Combination)*

To be taken for swelling pain in the throat, inflammation, and congestion.

V. Hoarsness

1. Mai-Men-Tung-Tang　　　　　麥門冬湯 [81]
(Ophiopogon Combination)

To be taken for severe cough and burning sensation in the throat.

2. Hsiang-Sheng-Po-Ti-Wan　　　響聲破笛丸 [108]
(Gasping Formula)

To be taken for hoarseness due to excessive singing and speaking.

MOUTH DISORDERS

I. Teeth

1. Ching-Wei-San　　　　　　　清胃散 [119]
(Coptis and Rehmannia Formula)
To be taken by those having a feeling of feverishness in the stomach and mouth, halitosis, coating on the tongue, toothache, gingivitis, pyorrhea, and bleeding gums.

2. Kuei-Chih-Wu-Wu-Tang　　　桂枝五物湯 [67]
(Cinnamon Five Herbs
Combination)
To be taken for gingivitis, decayed teeth, pyorrhea, swelling, pain, and redness. In cases involving constipation, add Rhubarb. In cases involving inflammation, add Fibrosum Gypsum.

II. Stomatitis

1. Kan-Lu-Yin　　　　　　　　甘露飲 [40]
(Sweet Combination)
To be taken for gingivitis, halitosis, stomatitis, and swelling pain in the throat.

CONDITIONS USUALLY TREATED BY SURGERY

I. Hemorrhoids and Prolapse of the Rectum

1. I-Tzu-Tang 乙字湯 [1]
(Cimicifuga Combinations)

This is a typical formula for hemorrhoidal bleeding, pain, anal fissure, and the initial stage of prolapse of the rectum. Those with a delicate constitution should take this formula with:

Szu-Wu-Tang 四物湯 [28]
(Tang-Kuei Four Combination)

2. Chiung-Kuei-Chiao-Ai-Tang 芎歸膠艾湯 [47]
(Capillaris and Gelatin Combination)

To be taken for continuous hemorrhoidal bleeding and resultant anemia.

3. Pu-Chung-I-Chi-Tang 補中益氣湯 [96]
(Ginseng and Astragalus Combination)

To be taken by those of delicate constitution with chills, poor complexion, stagnant blood, muscle atony with the symptoms of hemorrhoids, prolapse of the rectum, and night sweats.

4. Tzu-Yun-Kao　　　　　　　　　紫雲膏 [120]
(Lithospermum Ointment)
It is effective for external injuries, chilblain, burns, and
hemorrhoids. It can promote granulation and has bactericidal
action.

II. Frigorism and Gangrene

1. Tang-Kuei-Szu-　　　當歸四逆加吳茱萸生薑湯 [100]
　Ni-Chia-Wu-Chu-Yu-Shen-Chiang-Tang
(Tang-Kuei, Evodia and Ginger Combination)
To be taken for cold hands and feet, weak pulse, and severe
chills. It is effective for chilblain and gangrene.

III. Enterocele

1. Kuei-Chih-Chia-Shao-Yao-Tang　　桂枝加芍藥湯 [70]
(Cinnamon and Peony
Combination)
To be taken for enterocele with abdominal swelling and pain.

2. Ta-Chien-Chung-Tang
(Major Zanthoxylum Combination)　　大建中湯 [14]
To be taken for gastrointestinal weakness, loss of appetite,
chills in the abdomen, and abdominal pain.

IV. Injuries

1. Tao-Ho-Chen-Chi-Tang　　　　桃核承氣湯 [72]
(Persica and Rhubarb
Combination)
To be taken for pain and swelling of injuries due to fighting,
and for constipation. If there is no constipation, the patient
should take Kuei-Chih-Fu-Ling-Wan (Cinnamon and Hoelen
Formula).

2. Chi-Li-San   七厘散 [111]
(Musk and Catechu Formula)
This is effective for external injuries, stagnant blood, and
generalized pain.

V. Carbuncle

1. Ko-Ken-Tang   葛根湯 [101]
(Pueraria Combination)
To be taken for carbuncles inflammation, swelling, severe
chills, and when there is fever.

2. Shih-Wei-Pai-Tu-San   十味敗毒散 [11]
*(Bupleurum and
Schizonepeta Formula)*
To be taken by those having a tendency towards developing
carbuncles.

3. Tuo-Li-Hsiao-Tu-Yin   托裏消毒飲 [42]
(Gleditschia Combination)
To be taken for suppuration, and for gland and muscular
inflammation.

PART II

A Discussion of Commonly Used Herbal Formulas

(The symbol * means that a herbal formula has been approved for use in medical facilities by the Department of Pharmaceutical Affairs, Ministry of Health and Welfare, Japan)

(The symbol ▲ means that a herbal formula has been approved for use in medical facilities by the National Health Administration, Republic of China)

EXPLANATION OF THE IMPORTANT FORMULAS

1. I-Tzu-Tang 乙字湯 *
Cimicifuga Combination)
Main Herbs:
Cimicifuga 1.5 grams, Tang-Kuei 6.0 grams, Rhubarb 1.0 grams, Bupleurum 5.0 grams, Scute 3.0 grams, Licorice 2.0 grams
Effects:
This is a typical formula for hemorrhoids and prolapse of the rectum. Frequent use of this formula can improve the liver function, increase blood circulation, relieve constipation, and have hemostatic and analgesic effects.
Uses:
Ache of hemorrhoids, bleeding, and primary prolapse of the rectum.

2. Jen-Sheng-Tang 人參湯 *
(Ginseng and Ginger Combination)
Main Herbs:
Ginseng, Licorice, Atractylodes, Ginger (3.0 grams for each of these)
Effects:
This is effective for poor complexion, cold limbs, and tendencies toward fatigue and diarrhea. Those with gastrointestinal weakness, malnutrition, and endocrine disorders should take this formula.

Uses:
Gastritis, gastroptosis, stomach distension, peptic ulcer, sialosis, toxemia of pregnancy, intercostal neuralgia, bleeding in those of weak confirmation, and hemoptysis.

3. Jen-Sheng-Yang-Yung-Tang 人參養榮湯 *
(Ginseng Nutritive Combination)
Main Herbs:
Ginseng 3.0 grams, Atractylodes 4.0 grams, Astragalus 2.5 grams, Licorice 1.5 grams, Citrus 2.5 grams, Cinnamon 2.5 grams, Tang-Kuei 4.0 grams, Paeonia 4.0 grams, Rehmannia 4.0 grams, Schizandra 1.5 grams, Hoelen 4.0 grams, Polygala 1.5 grams.
Effects:
This is effective for those of delicate constitution with anemia, pallor, amnesia, insomnia, palpitations, and loss of appetite.
Uses:
Weakness, tuberculosis, amnesia, alopecia.

4. Jen-Sheng-Pai-Tu-San 人參敗毒散
(Ginseng and Mentha Formula)
Main Herbs:
Ginseng 2.0 grams, Qianghuo 2.0 grams, Tuhuo 2.0 grams, Bupleurum 2.0 grams, Peucedanum 2.0 grams, Cnidium 2.0 grams, Chih-Ko 2.0 grams, Platycodon 2.0 grams, Hoelen 2.0 grams, Licorice 1.0 grams, Mentha 1.0 grams, Ginger 1.0 grams.
Effects:
This formula is good for neck stiffness and pain in the limbs.
Uses:
Common cold, influenza, cough, nasal congestion, urticaria, and eczema.

5. Chi-Wu-Chiang-Hsia-Tang 七物降下湯 *
(Tang-Kuei and Gambir Combination)
Main Herbs:

Tang-Kuei 3.0 grams, Paeonia 3.0 grams, Rehmannia 3.0 grams, Cnidium 3.0 grams, Phellodendron 2.0 grams, Astragalus 3.0 grams, Gambir 2.0 grams.
Effects:
This is effective for those of weak confirmation with hypertension or kidney disorder.
Uses:
Essential and renal hypertension, chronic nephritis, and arteriosclerosis.

6. Pa-Wei-Tai-Hsia-Fang 八味帶下方
(Tang-Kuei and Eight Herbs Formula)
Main Herbs:
Smilax 4.0 grams, Tang-Kuei 5.0 grams, Cnidium 3.0 grams, Akebia 3.0 grams, Hoelen 3.0 grams, Citrus 2.0 grams, Lonicera 1.0 grams, Rhubarb 1.0 grams.
Effects:
As a leucorrhea agent, it is used for moderate inflammation and congestion, subacute or chronic leucorrhea.
Uses:
Leucorrhea with malodorous, purulent discharge with bad odor, and gonococci leucorrhea due to gonorrhea.

7. Pa-Wei-Ti-Huang-Wan 八味地黃丸 *
(Rehmannia Eight Formula)
Main Herbs:
Rehmannia 8.0 grams, Dioscorea 4.0 grams, Cornus 4.0 grams, Hoelen 3.0 grams, Moutan 3.0 grams, Alisma 3.0 grams, Cinnamon 1.0 grams, Aconite 1.0 grams.
Effects:
This is a well-known formula for kidney weakness which effectively increases vigor in people past middle age and in the elderly. It is especially effective for impotence, diabetes, and pruritis in the elderly.
Uses:
Diabetes, hypertension, neurasthenia, skin diseases with pruritis, cataract, and cystitis.

8. Chiu-Ping-Wu-Fu-Tang　九檳吳茯湯
(Areca Combination)
Main Herbs:
Areca Seed 4.0 grams, Magnolia Bark 3.0 grams, Cinnamon 3.0 grams, Citrus 3.0 grams, Ginger 3.0 grams, Rhubarb 1.0 grams, Inula 1.0 grams, Perilia 2.0 grams, Licorice 1.0 grams, Evodia 1.0 grams, Hoelen 3.0 grams.
Effects:
This formula is good for beriberi and relieves edema, rapid respiration, and generalized fatigue.
Uses:
Beriberi.

9. Shih-Chuan-Ta-Pu-Tang 十全大補湯　　　　▲*
(Ginseng and Tang-Kuei 10 Combination)
Main Herbs:
Ginseng 3.0 grams, Atractylodes 3.0 grams, Hoelen 3.0 grams, Cnidium 3.0 grams, Rehmannia 3.0 grams, Paeonia 3.0 grams, Cinnamon 3.0 grams, Tang-Kuei 3.0 grams, Astragalus 3.0 grams, Licorice 1.0 grams.
Effects:
This is a well-known tonic effective for chronic disease involving debility, anemia, loss of appetite, and dry skin.
Uses:
As a tonic after sickness, surgery, and childbirth; also for articular rheumatism, chilled tumor, and general debility.

10. Shih-Shen-Tang 十神湯　　　　　　　　　▲
(M.H. and Cimicifuga Combination)
Main Herbs:
Cnidium 3.0 grams, Licorice 3.0 grams, M.H. 3.0 grams, Perilla 3.0 grams, Angelica 3.0 grams, Cimicifuga 3.0 grams, Citrus 3.0 grams, Paeonia 3.0 grams, Pueraria 6.0 grams, Cyperus 3.0 grams, Ginger 2.0 grams, Jujube 2.0 grams.
Effects:
This is effective for the common cold with headache, fever without sweat, severe chill, and cough.

Uses:
Common cold.

11. Shih-Wei-Pai-Tu-San 十味散毒散 *
(Bupleurum and Schizonepeta Formula)
Main Herbs:
Bupleurum 3.0 grams, Cherrybark 3.0 grams, Platycodon 3.0 grams, Cnidium 3.0 grams, Hoelen 3.0 grams, Tuhuo 2.0 grams, Siler 2.0 grams, Licorice 1.0 grams, Ginger 1.0 grams, Schizonepeta 1.0 grams.
Effects:
This is a famous oral medication for skin diseases. The formula should be taken frequently in order to strengthen the liver, increase resistance of those with delicate constitution, and adjust any imbalance between autonomic nervous system and internal secretions.
Uses:
Urticaria, exzema, athlete's foot, furuncle.

12. San-Huang-Hsieh-Hsin-Tang 三黃瀉心湯或三黃錠 *
(Coptis and Rhubarb Combination)
San-Huang-Ting
(Coptis and Rhubarb Tablet)
Main Herbs:
Rhubarb 2.0 grams, Scute 1.0 grams, Coptis 1.0 grams.
Effects:
This is effective for those prone to stroke, fever, irritability, and insomnia. It is most effective for habitual constipation, and prevention of stroke.
Uses:
Stroke, hypertension, insomnia, habitual constipation, hemoptysis, nosebleed, and uterine bleeding.

13. Chuan-Chiung-Cha-Tiao-San 川芎茶調散 ▲ *
(Cnidium and Tea Formula)
Main Herbs:
Mentha 2.0 grams, Cnidium 3.0 grams, Schizonepeta 2.0

grams, Qianghuo 2.0 grams, Angelica 2.0 grams, Licorice 1.5 grams, Siler 2.0 grams, Tea 1.5 grams, Cyperus 4.0 grams.
Effects:
It is effective for vertigo, a feeling of heaviness in the head, headache, and migraine.
Uses:
Common cold, headache, and nasal congestion.

14. Ta-Chien-Chung-Tang　大建中湯　　　　　*
(Major Zanthoxylum Combination)
Main Herbs:
Zanthoxylum 2.0 grams, Ginseng 3.0 grams, Ginger 5.0 grams, Maltose 2.0 grams.
Effects:
To be taken by those of weak and chill confirmation with enteric palpitation with severe abdominal pain.
Uses:
Intestinal hernia, abdominal ache due to ascariasis, and localized peritonitis.

15. Ta-Chai-Hu-Tang　大柴胡湯　　　　　　*
(Major Bupleurum Combination)
Main Herbs:
Bupleurum 6.0 grams, Scute 3.0 grams, Paeonia 3.0 grams, Ginger 4.0 grams, Chih-Shih 2.0 grams, Jujube 3.0 grams, Rhubarb 1.0 grams, Pinellia 3.0 grams.
Effects:
It is effective for those of strong physique after middle age who experience insomnia, fatigue, lassitude, and loss of vigor.
Uses:
Gallstones, cholecystitis, lassitude, hepatitis, gastritis, hypertension, obesity, and habitual constipation.

16. Ta-Huang-Mu-Tan-Pi-Tang 大黄牡丹皮湯　　*
(Rhubarb and Moutan Combination)

Main Herbs:
Rhubarb 2.0 grams, Moutan 4.0 grams, Benincasa 6.0 grams, Mirabilium 4.0 grams, Persica 4.0 grams.
Effects:
This is good for stagnant blood, inflammation and suppuration within the lower body, especially in the lower abdomen. It is also effective for those whose vitality is good but who have a tendency towards constipation.
Uses:
Appendicitis, myoma of uterus, difficult menstruation, ovaritis, and pyelitis.

17. Hsiao-Pan-Hsia-Chia-Fu-Ling-Tang   *
(Pinellia and Hoelen Combination) 小半夏加茯苓湯
Main Herbs:
Pinellia 8.0 grams, Hoelen 5.0 grams, Ginger 1.0 grams.
Effects:
This is a common formula for vomiting in pregnancy or for other reasons.
Uses:
Toxemia of pregnancy, and vomiting.

18. Hsiao-Ching-Lung-Tang   小青龍湯   *
(Minor Blue Dragon Combination)
Main Herbs:
M.H. 3.0 grams, Paeonia 3.0 grams, Cinnamon 3.0 grams, Licorice 3.0 grams, Ginger 3.0 grams, Pinellia 6.0 grams, Schizandra 3.0 grams, Asarum 3.0 grams.
Effects:
This formula is effective for cough and wheezing due to the common cold or bronchitis. It is also effective for watery sputum and for promoting smooth bowel evacuation.
Uses:
Common cold, allergic rhinitis, bronchitis, bronchial asthma, lacrimation.

19. Hsiao-Chai-Hu-Tang 小柴胡湯 *
(Minor Bupleurum Combination)
Main Herbs:
Bupleurum 7.0 grams, Scute 3.0 grams, Ginseng 3.0 grams, Ginger 4.0 grams, Pinellia 5.0 grams, Jujube 3.0 grams, Licorice 2.0 grams.
Effects:
This is good to treat loss of appetite with fatigue, white coating on the tongue, or nausea.
Uses:
Common cold or other febrile diseases, bronchitis, gastritis, hepatitis, lymphadenitis, tuberculosis, and pleurisy.

20. Hsiao-Chien-Chung-Tang 小建中湯 *
(Minor Cinnamon and Peony Combination)
Main Herbs:
Paeonia 6.0 grams, Cinnamon 4.0 grams, Licorice 4.0 grams, Jujube 4.0 grams, Maltose 20 grams, Ginger 2.0 grams.
Effects:
This formula is good for children of delicate constitution. Its frequent use can improve general health and increase brain function. It is also effective for bed-wetting, night crying, stomach ache, and hernia. It is especially good for constipation in preschool children.
Uses:
As a tonic for children with delicate constitution; to treat bedwetting, hernia, gastritis, and nervous stomach ache.

21. Mu-Fang-Chi-Tang 木防己湯
(Stephania and Ginseng Combination)
Main Herbs:
Stephania 4.0 grams, Cinnamon 3.0 grams, Ginseng 3.0 grams, Gypsum 10 grams.
Effects:
This formula is good to treat a feeling of hardness beneath the

heart, heart disorder with edema, and difficulty in urination.
Uses:
Valvular disease, cardiac asthma, and nephritis.

22. Fen-Hsiao-Tang 分消湯 *
(Hoelen and Alisma Combination)
Main Herbs:
Atractylodes 5.0 grams, Hoelen 2.5 grams, Citrus 2.0 grams,
Magnolia bark 2.0 grams, Cyperus 2.0 grams, Polyporus 2.0
grams, Alisma 2.0 grams, Areca 1.0 grams, Cardamon 1.0
grams, Inula 1.0 grams, Ginger 1.0 grams, Juncus 1.0 grams,
Chih-Shih 1.0 grams.
Effects:
This formula is used to ease breathing, stagnation, and edema.
To be taken in the initial stage of ascites when good vigor is
present.
Uses:
Nephritis, renal necrosis, ascites, peritonitis, cirrhosis.

23. Liu-Wei-Ti-Huang-Wan 六味地黃丸 ▲*
(Rehmannia Six Formula)
Main Herbs:
Rehmannia 6.0 grams, Cornus 3.0 grams, Dioscorea 3.0
grams, Alisma 3.0 grams, Moutan 3.0 grams, Hoelen 3.0
grams.
Effects:
This formula is good for aching near the waist and feet,
vertigo, spermatorrhea, and polyuria due to renal weakness.
To be used for milder symptoms than those of Pa-Wei-Ti-
Huang-Wan (Rehmannia Eight Formula).
Uses:
Diabetes, senile diseases, impotence, spermatorrhea, and
nephritis.

24. Liu-Chun-Tzu-Tang 六君子湯 ▲*
(Major Six Herbs Combination)

Main Herbs:
Ginseng 4.0 grams, Atractylodes 4.0 grams, Hoelen 4.0 grams, Pinellia 4.0 grams, Citrus 2.0 grams, Ginger 2.0 grams, Jujube 2.0 grams, Licorice 1.0 grams.
Effects:
To be taken by the patient with gastrointestinal weakness, gastric stagnation, loss of appetite, vomiting, anemia, and tendency towards fatigue.
Uses:
Gastrectasis, gastroptosis, chronic gastroenteritis, and delicate constitution.

25. Tien-Wang-Pu-Hsin-Tan 天王補心丹 ▲
(Ginseng and Zizyphus Formula)
Main Herbs:
Rehmannia 1.3 grams, Ginseng 1.3 grams, Scrophularia 1.3 grams, Salvia 1.3 grams, Hoelen 1.3 grams, Platycodon 1.3 grams, Polygal 1.3 grams, Biota 1.3 grams, Asparagus 1.3 grams, Ophiopogon 1.3 grams, Tang-Kuei 1.3 grams, Schizandra 1.3 grams, Anemone 1.3 grams, Cinnabar 1.3 grams, Zizyphus 1.3 grams.
Effects:
This formula is effective for mental exhaustion, emotional instability, spermatorrhea and amnesia.
Uses:
Constipation, insomnia, and amnesia.

26. Wu-Ling-San 五苓散 *
(Hoelen Five Herbs Formula)
Main Herbs:
Hoelen 6.5 grams, Alisma 6.0 grams, Polyporus 4.5 grams, Cinnamon 3.0 grams, Atractylodes 4.5 grams.
Effects:
This formula is good for 'watery' endocrine disorders such as those indicated by thirst, oliguria, headache, nausea, vomiting, and intoxication.

Uses:
Common cold of infants, intoxication, nephritis, and renal necrosis.

27. Szu-Chun-Tzu-Tang 四君子湯 *
(Major Four Herbs Combination)
Main Herbs:
Ginseng 4.0 grams, Atractylodes 4.0 grams, Hoelen 4.0 grams, Licorice 1.5 grams, Ginger 1.5 grams, Jujube 1.5 grams.
Effects:
To be taken for lack of vigor, gastrointestinal weakness, and anemia. Frequent use of this formula can increase the functions of the spleen and stomach function.
Uses:
Delicate digestion, gastroptosis, and gastric ulcer.

28. Szu-Wu-Tang 四物湯 ▲*
(Tang-Kuei Four Combination)
Main Herbs:
Rehmannia 4.0 grams, Tang-Kuei 4.0 grams, Cnidium 4.0 grams, Paeonia 4.0 grams.
Effects:
This formula is good to treat female disorders, and to be used as a body and blood tonic.
Uses:
Disorders before or after childbirth, menstrual irregularity, infertility, chilblain, and menopausal disorders.

29. Pai-Hu-Chia-Jen-Sheng-Tang 白虎加人參湯 *
(Ginseng and Gypsum Combination)
Main Herbs:
Gypsum 15 grams, Anemarrhena 5.0 grams, Oryza 10 grams, Licorice 2.0 grams, Ginseng 3.0 grams.

Effects:
This formula is effective for febrile diseases and thirst.
Uses:
Acute fever, sunstroke, diabetes, and eczema.

30. Pan-Hsia-Hou-Pu-Tang 半夏厚朴湯 *
(Pinellia and Magnolia Combination)
Main Herbs:
Pinellia 6.0 grams, Magnolia bark 3.0 grams, Hoelen 5.0 grams, Perillia 2.0 grams, Ginger 4.0 grams.
Effects:
This formula is good for neurosis, nervousness, and emotional instability.
Uses:
Neurasthenia, neurosis, bronchitis, and bronchial asthma.

31. Pan-Hsia-Pai-Chu-Tien-Ma-Tang 半夏白朮天麻湯 *
(Pinellia and Gastrodia Combination)
Main Herbs:
Pinellia 3.0 grams, Atractylodes 3.0 grams, Citrus 3.0 grams, Hoelen 3.0 grams, Malt 2.0 grams, Gastrodia 2.0 grams, Ginger 2.0 grams, Shen-Chu 2.0 grams, Astragalus 1.5 grams, Ginseng 1.5 grams, Alisma 1.5 grams, Phellodendron 1.0 grams.
Effects:
This formula is good for the spleen and stomach. It is effective for those of delicate constitution with gastrointestinal weakness, recurrent headaches, and vertigo.
Uses:
Gastric distension, gastroptosis, gastritis, neurosis, hypertension, and suppuration.

32. Pan-Hsia-Hsieh-Hsin-Tang 半夏瀉心湯 *
(Pinellia Combination)

Main Herbs:
Pinellia 6.0 grams, Scute 3.0 grams, Coptis 1.0 grams, Ginseng 3.0 grams, Jujube 3.0 grams, Ginger 3.0 grams, Licorice 3.0 grams.

Effects:
This formula and An-Chung-San (Cardamon and Fennel Formula) are two famous formulas for gastrointestinal diseases. It is effective for those having borborygmus, diarrhea, gastritis, gastroptosis, constipation, nausea, and vomiting.

Uses:
Gastroenteritis, gastrectasis, gastroptosis, and gastric ulcer.

33. Pan-Hsieh-Liu-Chun-Tzu-Tang 半瀉六君子湯
(Pinellia and Ginseng Six Combination)
Main Herbs:
Ginseng 4.0 grams, Atractylodes 4.0 grams, Hoelen 4.0 grams, Licorice 1.0 grams, Pinellia 4.0 grams, Citrus 2.0 grams, Ginger 1.0 grams, Scute 3.0 grams, Coptis 3.0 grams, Ostrea testa 4.0 grams.

Effects:
It is effective for stomach distension, vomiting, stomach-ache, and malnutrition.

Uses:
Gastroenteritis, gastric ulcer, gastroptosis, and delicate constitution.

34. Shen-Chiang-Hsieh-Hsin-Tang 生薑瀉心湯 *
(Pinellia and Ginger Combination)
Main Herbs:
Pinellia 5.0 grams, Scute 3.0 grams, Licorice 3.0 grams, Ginseng 3.0 grams, Ginger 4.0 grams, Jujube 3.0 grams, Coptis 1.0 grams.

Effects:
To be taken for symptoms similar to those of Pan-Hsia-Hsieh-Hsin-Tang (Pinellia Combination), and for halitosis.

Uses:
Gastroenteritis, acid stomach, and fermentative diarrhea.

35. Shen-Hua-Tang 生化湯 ▲
(Tang-Kuei and Ginger Combination)
Main Herbs:
Tang-Kuei 5.0 grams, Cnidium 5.0 grams, Persica 3.0 grams, Ginger 2.0 grams, Licorice 2.0 grams.
Effects:
This is a good postpartum formula. Frequent use of this formula can nourish the body and dispel stagnant blood.
Uses:
As a tonic for the blood, for abdominal ache, and for postpartum bleeding.

36. Chia-Wei-Hsiao-Yao-San 加味逍遙散 *
(Bupleurum and Peony Formula)
Main Herbs:
Tang-Kuei 3.0 grams, Paeonia 3.0 grams, Atractylodes 3.0 grams, Hoelen 3.0 grams, Bupleurum 3.0 grams, Licorice 2.0 grams, Moutan 2.0 grams, Gardenia 2.0 grams, Ginger 1.0 grams, Mentha 1.0 grams.
Effects:
This formula is good to treat climacteric disturbances, menstrual irregularity, and various symptoms due to abortion or salpingotomy. These symptoms may include emotional instability, nagging, a tendency towards fatigue, headache, constipation, and lumbago.
Uses:
Menstrual irregularity, blood diseases, hysteria, and menopausal disorder.

37. Ping-Wei-San 平胃散 ▲*
(Magnolia and Ginger Formula)

64

Main Herbs:
Atractylodes 4.0 grams, Magnolia bark 3.0 grams, Citrus 3.0 grams, Ginger 1.0 grams, Jujube 2.0 grams, Licorice 1.0 grams.
Effects:
It is effective for stomach and intestinal disturbances due to indigestion, and for borborygmus and diarrhea after eating.
Uses:
Gastritis, indigestion, and loss of appetite.

38. Kan-Mai-Ta-Tsao-Tang 甘麥大棗湯 *
(Licorice and Jujube Combination)
Main Herbs:
Licorice 3.0 grams, Jujube 2.5 grams, Wheat 14 grams.
Effects:
This formula is good to treat nervousness, hysteria, insomnia, emotional instability, and frequent yawning.
Uses:
Hysteria, chorea, night crying, and epilepsy.

39. Kan-Tsao-Hsieh-Hsin-Tang 甘草瀉心湯 *
(Pinellia and Licorice Combination)
Main Herbs:
Pinellia 5.0 grams, Scute 2.5 grams, Ginger 2.5 grams, Ginseng 2.5 grams, Zizyphus 2.5 grams, Licorice 2.5 grams, Coptis 1.0 grams.
Effects:
To be taken for symptoms similar to those treated by Pan-Hsia-Hsieh-Hsin-Tang (Pinellia Combination) when there is also emotional instability.
Uses:
Gastroenteritis, severe diarrhea, and insomnia.

40. Kan-Lu-Yin 甘露飲 ▲
(Sweet Combination)

Main Herbs:
Rehmannia 4.0 grams, Asparagus 2.0 grams, Ophiopogon 2.0 grams, Dendrobium 2.0 grams, Chih-Shih 2.0 grams, Capillaris 2.0 grams, Scute 2.0 grams, Eriobotrya 2.0 grams, Licorice 2.0 grams.

Effects:
This formula is good for moist fever in the digestive system with swelling and suppuration in the tongue, gingiva, and throat.

Uses:
Gingivitis, pyorrhea, stomatitis, and scurvy.

41. An-Chung-San 安中散 ▲*
(Cardamon and Fennel Formula)

Main Herbs:
Cardamon 1.0 grams, Fennel 1.5 grams, Cinnamon 4.0 grams, Corydalis 3.0 grams, Ostrea testa 3.0 grams, Licorice .5 grams, Galanga 0.5 grams.

Effects:
This is effective for those subject to chill confirmation, gastrointestinal discomfort, and nausea. It is given to those of delicate constitution who have a fondness for sweet food. This formula contains no soda and is good for those who become toxic by taking soda for a long time.

Uses:
Gastroenteritis, gastritis, acid stomach, and chronic stomachache.

42. Tuo-Li-Hsiao-Tu-Yin 托裏消毒飲
(Gleditschia Combination)

Main Herbs:
Ginseng 3.0 grams, Cnidium 3.0 grams, Platycodon 3.0 grams, Atractylodes 3.0 grams, Paeonia 3.0 grams, Tang-Kuei 5.0 grams, Hoelen 5.0 grams, Gleditschia 2.0 grams, Angelica 1.0 grams, Astragalus 1.5 grams, Lonicera 1.5 grams, Licorice 1.0 grams.

Effects:
This formula is good for suppurative diseases. Those of delicate constitution should take Chien-Chin-Nei-Tuo-San (Astragalus and Platycodon Formula).
Uses:
Suppurative lymphadenitis, subcutaneous suppuration, carbuncle, and periproctitis.

43. Fang-Chi-Huang-Chi-Tang 防己黃耆湯 *
(Stephania and Astragalus Combination)
Main Herbs:
Stephania 5.0 grams, Astragalus 5.0 grams, Atractylodes 3.0 grams, Ginger 3.0 grams, Jujube 3.0 grams, Licorice 1.5 grams.
Effects:
To be taken by those of obese constitution with a tendency towards fatigue and perspiration, and who suffer from arthrorheumatism, muscle pain, and gout. It is especially effective for women.
Uses:
Ephidrosis, rheumatism, arthritis, and obesity.

44. Fang-Feng-Tung-Sheng-San 防風通聖散 *
(Siler and Platycodon Formula)
Main Herbs:
Siler 1.2 grams, Schizonepeta 1.2 grams, Forsythia 1.2 grams, M.H. 1.2 grams, Mentha 1.2 grams, Cnidium 1.2 grams, Tang-Kuei 1.2 grams, Paeonia 1.2 grams, Atractylodes 2.0 grams, Gardenia 1.2 grams, Rhubarb 1.5 grams, Mirabilitum 1.5 grams, Gypsum 2.0 grams, Scute 2.0 grams, Platycodon 2.0 grams, Licorice 2.0 grams, Talcum 3.0 grams, Ginger 1.2 grams.
Effects:
This formula is good for treating constipation in those with an obese constitution.

Uses:
Obesity, habitual constipation, heart trouble, arteriosclerosis, stroke, and nephritis.

45. I-Kan-San 抑肝散 *
(Bupleurum Formula)
Main Herbs:
Tang-Kuei 3.0 grams, Gambir 3.0 grams, Cnidium 3.0 grams, Atractylodes 4.0 grams, Hoelen 4.0 grams, Bupleurum 2.0 grams, Licorice 1.5 grams.
Effects:
This is good to treat liver disease, and is effective for "internal heat," nervousness, irritability, and insomnia.
Uses:
Neurosis, epilepsy, hysteria, night crying, insomnia, and neuro-shoulder stiffness.

46. Shao-Yao-Kan-Tsao-Tang 芍藥甘草湯 *
(Peony and Licorice Combination)
Main Herbs:
Paeonia 6.0 grams, Licorice 6.0 grams.
Effects:
It is effective for rapid clonic convulsion, pain in the limbs, and colic of kidney stones and gallstones.
Uses:
Convulsion of the hands and feet after strenuous exercises, abdominal ache due to gall or kidney stones, and pain due to difficult menstruation.

47. Chiung-Kuei-Chiao-Ai-Tang 芎歸膠艾湯 *
(Tang-Kuei and Gelatin Combination)
Main Herbs:
Tang-Kuei 4.0 grams, Cnidium 3.0 grams, Paeonia 4.0 grams, Licorice 3.0 grams, Artemisia leaves 3.0 grams, Rehmannia 5.0 grams, Gelatin 3.0 grams.

Effects:
This formula is good to treat anemia due to bleeding.
Uses:
Uterine bleeding, hemorrhoidal bleeding, prevention of abortion, and hematuria.

48. Wu-Chu-Yu-Tang、吳茱萸湯 *
(Evodia Combination)
Main Herbs:
Evodia 4.0 grams, Ginseng 3.0 grams, Jujube 3.0 grams, Ginger 6.0 grams.
Effects:
This formula is good for "cool stomach," chills, vomiting, and diarrhea. It is also effective for stagnant water in the stomach, a feeling of fullness beneath the heart, vomiting, and headache.
Uses:
Migraine, habitual headache, and hiccough.

49. Hsin-I-Ching-Fei-Tang 辛夷清肺湯 *
(Magnolia and Gypsum Combination)
Main Herbs:
Magnolia flower 2.0 grams, Eriobotrya 2.0 grams, Anemarrhena 3.0 grams, Lily 3.0 grams, Scute 3.0 grams, Gypsum 5.0 grams, Ophiopogon 5.0 grams, Gardenia 3.0 grams, Cimicifuga 1.0 grams.
Effects:
This formula is good to treat lung fever, nasal congestion, nasal fever, and thirst.
Uses:
Nasal discharge, rhinorrhea and rhinitis.

50. Chin-Sou-Ku-Ching-Wan 金鎖固精丸 ▲*
(Lotus Stamen Combination)

Main Herbs:
Tribulus 5.0 grams, Euryale 5.0 grams, Lotus stamen 5.0 grams, Dragon-bone 2.5 grams, Ostrea testa 2.5 grams.
Effects:
This formula is good for nourishing the body and for nervous exhaustion.
Uses:
Nocturnal emission, spermatorrhea, bed-wetting and sexual neurasthenia.

51. Chih-Kan-Tsao-Tang 炙甘草湯   *
(Licorice Combination)
Main Herbs:
Licorice 3.0 grams, Jujube 3.0 grams, Gelatin 2.0 grams, Ginger 3.0 grams, Ginseng 3.0 grams, Rehmannia 6.0 grams, Cinnaomon 3.0 grams, Ophiopogon 6.0 grams, Cannabis seed 3.0 grams.
Effects:
This is effective for palpitations, gasping, stagnant pulse, and improving delicate constitution.
Uses:
Heart trouble, palpitation, hypertension, and goiter.

52. Ting-Chuan-San 定喘散   ▲
(M.H. and Ginkgo Combination)
Main Herbs:
Ginkgo 3.0 grams, M.H. 1.0 grams, Pinellia 2.0 grams, Tussilago 3.0 grams, Morus 3.0 grams, Perilla fruit 3.0 grams, Almond 3.0 grams, Scute 3.0 grams, Licorice 2.0 grams, Ginger 1.0 grams.
Effects:
This is a common formula commonly used to treat asthma. It is effective for cough, asthma, excessive sputum, emotional instability, and loss of appetite.
Uses:
Bronchitis and bronchial asthma.

70

53. Shiang-Su-San 香蘇散
(Cyperus and Perilla Formula)
Main Herbs:
Cyperus 3.5 grams, Perilla 1.5 grams, Citrus 3.0 grams, Licorice 1.0 grams, Ginger 1.0 grams.
Effects:
To be taken for mild cases of the common cold, a feeling of hardness beneath the heart, anxiety due to stress, and stomach disorders.
Uses:
Mild cases of the common cold, nervous exhaustion, and food poisoning due to fish or meat.

54. Ling-Kuei-Chu-Kan-Tang 苓桂朮甘湯   *
(Atractylodes and Hoelen Combination)
Main Herbs:
Hoelen 6.0 grams, Cinnamon 4.0 grams, Atractylodes 3.0 grams, Licorice 2.0 grams.
Effects:
This formula is good for increasing brain function, and for treating vertigo, a feeling of heaviness in the head, tinnitus, and gasping. It is especially effective for vertigo accompanied by chronic headache.
Uses:
Palpitation, neurosis, tinnitus, insomnia, and temporary nearsightedness.

55. Ling-Kan-Chiang-Wei-Hsin-Hsia-Jen-Tang
(Hoelen and Schizandra Combination) 苓甘薑味辛夏仁湯
Main Herbs:
Hoelen 4.0 grams, Licorice 2.0 grams, Ginger 2.0 grams, Schizandra 3.0 grams, Pinellia 4.0 grams, Asarum 2.0 grams, Almond 4.0 grams.
Effects:
This is effective for those of delicate constitution with asthmatic wheezing and cough, especially for when it is due to

71

chronic bronchitis of the elderly and emphysema.
Uses:
Emphysema, bronchial asthma, cardiac asthma, and chronic nephritis.

56. Hsi-Kan-Ming-Mu-Tang 洗肝明目湯 ▲
(Gardenia and Vitex Combination)
Main Herbs:
Tang-Kuei 1.5 grams, Paeonia 1.5 grams, Cnidium 1.5 grams, Rehmannia 1.5 grams, Scute 1.5 grams, Gardenia 1.5 grams, Forsythia 1.5 grams, Siler 1.5 grams, Cassia Seed 1.5 grams, Coptis 1.0 grams, Schizonepeta 1.0 grams, Metha 1.0 grams, Qianghuo 1.0 grams, Vitex 1.0 grams, Chrysanthemum 1.0 grams, Gypsum 3.0 grams, Platycodon 1.0 grams, Licorice 1.0 grams, Tribulus 1.0 grams.
Effects:
It is mainly used by those of the firm and febrile type with eye disorders, inflammation, congestion, keratitis, and conjuctivitis.
Uses:
Hardened corneas, keratitis, conjunctivitis, and iritis.

57. Pao-Chan-Wu-Yu-Fang 保産無憂方 (安胎飲) ▲
(An-Tai-Yin)
(Tang-Kuei and Parsley Combination)
Main Herbs:
Magnolia bark 1.0 grams, Artemisia leaves 1.0 grams, Cnidium 3.0 grams, Tang-Kuei 3.0 grams, Schizonepeta 1.0 grams, Fritillary 2.0 grams, Cuscuta 3.0 grams, Qianghuo 1.0 grams, Licorice 1.0 grams, Chih-Ko 1.0 grams, Paeonia 2.0 grams, Ginger 1.0 grams, Astragalus 1.0 grams.
Effects:
The common name of this formula is Shih-San-Wei (Thirteen-in-One-Formula or An-Tai-Yin). It is an effective tonic for the body and blood.

Uses:
Vomiting during pregnancy, watery sputum, waist ache, abdominal pain, premature contractions, and frequent bleeding.

58. Shen-Mi-Tang　神秘湯　　　　　　　*
(M.H. and Magnolia Combination)
Main Herbs:
M.H. 5.0 grams, Perilla 1.5 grams, Citrus 2.5 grams, Magnolia bark 3.0 grams, Licorice 2.0 grams, Bupleurum 2.0 grams, Almond 4.0 grams.
Effects:
This formula is good for difficult breathing, with a moderate amount of sputum.
Uses:
Bronchial asthma in children or adults.

59. Chai-Hu-Kuei-Chih-Tang 柴胡桂枝湯　　　*
(Bupleurum and Cinnamon Combination)
Main Herbs:
Bupleurum 5.0 grams, Pinellia 4.0 grams, Licorice 1.5 grams, Cinnamon 2.5 grams, Scute 2.0 grams, Ginseng 2.0 grams, Paeonia 2.5 grams, Jujube 2.0 grams, Ginger 1.0 grams.
Effects:
This is a combined formula of Hsiao-Chai-Hu-Tang (Minor Bupleurum Combination) and Kuei-Chih-Tang (Cinnamon Combination).
It is effective for a lingering cold, fever, and pressing sensation at the chest and the abdomen. It is also effective for severe pain and loss of appetite due to gastrointestinal discomfort.
Uses:
Common cold, pleurisy, severe stomach ache, and loss of appetite.

柴胡桂枝乾薑湯
60. Chai-Hu-Kuei-Chih-Kan-Chiang-Tang　　*
(Bupleurum, Cinnamon and Ginger Combination)

Main Herbs:
Bupleurum 6.0 grams, Cinnamon 3.0 grams, Trichosanthes Root 3.0 grams, Scute 3.0 grams, Ostrea testa 3.0 grams, Ginger 2.0 grams, Licorice 2.0 grams.

Effects:
It is effective for those of delicate constitution with pallor, mild fever, cough, insomnia, palpitation, and diarrhea.

Uses:
Common cold, nervous exhaustion, insomnia, and wheezing and palpitations.

61. Chai-Ko-Chiai-Chi-Tang　柴葛解肌湯　　▲
(Bupleurum and Pueraria Combination)

Main Herbs:
Bupleurum 4.0 grams, Pueraria 4.0 grams, Scute 3.0 grams, Paeonia 3.0 grams, Qianghuo 2.0 grams, Angelica 2.0 grams, Platycodon 2.0 grams, Licorice 2.0 grams, Jujube 2.0 grams, Gypsum 5.0 grams, Ginger 1.0 gram.

Effects:
The patient having common cold or influenza, but who has not been cured by Ma-Huang-Tang (M.H. Combination), Kuei-Chih-Tang (Cinnamon Combination), and Ko-Ken-Tang (Pueraria Combination) should take this formula. It is also taken for thirst and for pain in the limbs.

Uses:
Common cold, pneumonia, and various fevers.

62. Chai-Hu-Chia-Lung-Ku-Mu-Li-Tang　　　　　*
(Bupleurum and Dragon-Bone Combination)

Main Herbs:　　　　　　　　柴胡加龍骨牡蠣湯
Bupleurum 5.0 grams, Pinellia 4.0 grams, Dragon-Bone 2.5 grams, Scute 2.5 grams, Ginger 2.5 grams, Cinnamon 3.0 grams, Hoelen 3.0 grams, Ostrea testa 2.5 grams, Jujube 2.5 grams, Rhubarb 1.0 grams, Ginseng 2.5 grams.

Effects:
This formula is good for improving health and increasing vigor. It increases mental stability, palpitations, and decreases insomnia, constipation, and vertigo. It is also an effective treatment for nervousness in children or for epilepsy.
Uses:
Arteriosclerosis, hypertension, habitual insomnia, kidney diseases, and epilepsy.

63. Chen-Wu-Tang 眞武湯
(Vitality Combination)
Main Herbs:
Hoelen 5.0 grams, Paeonia 3.0 grams, Atractylodes 3.0 grams, Ginger 3.0 grams, Aconite 1.0 grams.
Effects:
This is a formula frequently used for diseases due to endocrine disorder. It is effective for sweats, vertigo, palpitations, chilling of the limbs, and diarrhea.
Uses:
Chronic diarrhea, gastrointestinal weakness, fever, peritonitis, and appendicitis.

64. Yin-Chen-Hao-Tang 茵陳蒿湯   *
(Capillaris Combination)
Main Herbs:
Capillaris 4.0 grams, Gardenia 3.0 grams, Rhubarb 1.0 grams.
Effects:
This is a popular formula for jaundice with chest distension, vomiting, thirst, and decreased urinary volume.
Uses:
Pneumonia, nephritis, renal nephrosis, and food poisoning.

65. Yin-Chen-Wu-Ling-San 茵陳五苓散   *
(Capillaris and Hoelen Five Formula)

Main Herbs:
Capillaris 4.0 grams, Cinnamon 3.0 grams, Polyporus 4.5 grams, Hoelen, 4.5 grams, Atractylodes 4.5 grams, Alisma 6.0 grams.

Effects:
This is a formula of Wu-Ling-San (Hoelen Five Herb Formula) and Capillaris Herba. It is effective for thirst, difficulty in urination, and a tendency towards liver disturbances or jaundice.

Uses: Pneumonia, nephritis, renal necrosis, and ascites.

66. Kuei-Chih-Fu-Ling-Wan 桂枝茯苓丸   *
(Cinnamon and Hoelen Formula)

Main Herbs:
Cinnamon 4.0 grams, Hoelen 4.0 grams, Moutan 4.0 grams, Persica 4.0 grams, Paeonia 4.0 grams.

Effects:
This formula is good for improving blood circulation. It will dispel stagnant blood, internal heat with chilling of the lower body, headache, aching shoulders, sore muscles, and menstrual irregularity.

Uses:
Disturbances due to menstrual irregularities, eczema, freckles, and internal bleeding due to injury.

67. Kuei-Chih-Wu-Wu-Tang 桂枝五物湯
(Cinnamon Five Herbs Combination)

Main Herbs:
Cinnamon 4.0 grams, Scute 4.0 grams, Rehmannia 4.0 grams, Hoelen 8.0 grams, Platycodon 3.0 grams.

Uses:
Toothache, gingivitis, stomatitis, and pyorrhea in those of strong confirmation.

68. Kuei-Chih-Chia-Chu-Fu-Tang 桂枝加朮附湯   *
(Cinnamon and Aconite Combination)

Main Herbs:
Cinnamon 4.0 grams, Paeonia 4.0 grams, Jujube 4.0 grams,
Ginger 4.0 grams, Licorice 2.0 grams, Atractylodes 4.0 grams,
Aconite 1.0 grams.
Effects:
This is a commonly used formula for chronic neuralgia and
rheumatism. It is also effective for aching and numbness in the
limbs or difficulty in bending at the waist.
Uses:
Neuralgia, arthritis, and rheumatism.

69. Kuei-Chih-Chia-Lung-Ku-Mu-Li-Tang   *
(Cinnamon and Dragon-Bone Combination)
Main Herbs: 桂枝加龍骨牡蠣湯
Cinnamon 4.0 grams, Paeonia 4.0 grams, Jujube 4.0 grams,
Ginger 4.0 grams, Licorice 2.0 grams, Licorice 2.0 grams,
Dragon-Bone 3.0 grams, Ostrea testa 3.0 grams.
Effects:
This formula is Kuei-Chih-Tang (Cinnamon Combination)
plus Dragon-Bone and Ostrea testa. To be taken by the patient
of delicate constitution with fatigue who is easily excitable and
feels fatigued.
Uses:
Neurosis, lack of vigor, and impotence.

70. Kuei-Chih-Chia-Shao-Yao-Tang   桂枝加芍藥湯   *
(Cinnamon and Paeonia Combination)
Main Herbs:
Cinnamon 4.0 grams, Paeonia 6.0 grams, Jujube 4.0 grams,
Ginger 4.0 grams, Licorice 2.0 grams.
Effects:
This formula is good for chills, abdominal distension and
pain, and diarrhea.
Uses:
Colitis, peritonitis, and proctitis.

71. Kuei-Chih-Chia-Huang-Chi-Tang　桂枝加黃耆湯
(Cinnamon and Astragalus Combination)
Main Herbs:
Cinnamon 4.0 grams, Paeonia 4.0 grams, Jujube 4.0 grams, Ginger 4.0 grams, Astragalus 3.0 grams.
Effects:
This formula is good for those with moist and atonic skin, night sweats, and numbness.
Uses:
Ephidrosis, otitis media, blisters, and skin diseases.

72. Tao-Ho-Chen-Chi-Tang　桃核承氣湯　　　　*
(Persica and Rhubarb Combination)
Main Herbs:
Persica 5.0 grams, Rhubarb 3.0 grams, Cinnamon 4.0 grams, Mirabilitum 2.0 grams, Licorice 1.5 grams.
Effects:
This is a well-known formula for stagnant blood, facial redness with darkness, headache, dizziness, chill in the lower abdomen, aching near the waist, constipation, menstrual irregularities, and scanty urination due to external injury.
Uses:
Habitual constipation, freckles, eczema, disturbance due to menstrual irregularities, menopausal disorders, and neuralgia.

73. Chin-Chieh-Lien-Chiao-Tang　荊芥連翹湯
(Schizonepeta and Forsythia Combination)
Main Herbs:
Tang-Kuei 2.0 grams, Paeonia 2.0 grams, Cnidium 2.0 grams, Scute 2.0 grams, Gardenia 2.0 grams, Forsythia 2.0 grams, Siler 2.0 grams, Schizonepeta 2.0 grams, Chih-Ko 2.0 grams, Platycodon 2.0 grams, Angelica 2.0 grams, Bupleurum 2.0 grams, Licorice 1.5 grams.
Effects:
This formula is good for otitis, rhinitis and suppuration. It is

also effective for those with dark skin and sweaty palms and feet.

Uses:
Glandular diseases of adolescence, otitis media, suppuration, and rhinitis.

74. Chin-Fang-Pai-Tu-San 荊防敗毒散
(Schizonepeta and Siler Formula)
Main Herbs:
Schizonepeta 1.5 grams, Siler 1.5 grams, Qianghuo 1.5 grams, Tuhuo 1.5 grams, Bupleurum 1.5 grams, Peucedanum 1.5 grams, Mentha 1.5 grams, Platycodon 1.5 grams, Forsythia 1.5 grams, Chih-Ko 1.5 grams, Cnidium 1.5 grams, Lonicera 1.5 grams, Licorice 1.0 grams, Ginger 1.5 grams.
Effects:
This formula is good to treat suppuration, onset of severe chill, fever, inflammation, swelling, and pain.
Uses:
Carbuncle, urticaria, eczema, scabies, "scald head," suppuration, and dermatitis.

75. Hsiao-Feng-San 消風散   *
(Tang-Kuei and Arctium Formula)
Main Herbs:
Tang-Kuei 3.0 grams, Rehmannia 3.0 grams, Gypsum 3.0 grams, Anemarrhena 1.5 grams, Sesame 1.5 grams, Atractylodes 2.0 grams, Arctium 2.0 grams, Siler 2.0 grams, Akebia 2.0 grams, Licorice 1.0 grams, Cicadae 1.0 grams, Sophora 1.0 gram, Schizonepeta 1.0 gram, Sesame 1.5 grams.
Effects:
This formula is good for skin diseases with internal heat, copious secretions, and pruritis. It is effective for eczema with sweat and for scabies.
Uses:
Chronic eczema and urticaria.

76. Ma-Tzu-Jen-Wan 麻子仁丸 *
(Almond and Cannabis Formula)
Main Herbs:
Cannabis Seed 5.0 grams, Paeonia 2.0 grams, Chih-Shih 2.0 grams, Magnolia bark 2.0 grams, Rhubarb 4.0 grams, Almond 2.0 grams.
Effects:
This is a moderate purgative. It is effective for constipation in the delicate and convalescent elderly.
Uses:
Habitual constipation and hemorrhoids due to constipation.

77. Ma-Hsing-Kan-Shih-Tang 麻杏甘石湯 *
(M.H. and Almond Combination)
Main Herbs:
M.H. 4.0 grams, Almond 4.0 grams, Licorice 2.0 grams, Gypsum 10.0 grams.
Effects:
This is a commonly used formula for bronchial asthma, especially in children. It is used to treat severe cough, with extreme thirst and perspiration on the forehead at onset.
Uses:
Bronchitis and bronchial asthma.

78. Ma-Hsing-I-Kan-Tang 麻杏薏甘湯 *
(M.H. and Coix Combination)
Main Herbs:
M.H. 4.0 grams, Almond 3.0 grams, Coix 10.0 grams, Licorice 2.0 grams.
Effects:
This is a broadly used formula for rheumatic pain.
Uses:
Rheumatic pain, arthritis, and neuralgia.

79. Ma-Huang-Tang 麻黃湯 *
(M.H. Combination)

Main Herbs:
M.H. 5.0 grams, Almond 5.0 grams, Cinnamon 4.0 grams, Licorice 1.5 grams.
Effects:
The main symptom treated by this formula is generalized ache without perspiration, but with wheezing and polyuria.
Uses:
Common cold, asthma, and rhinitis.

80. Ma-Huang-Hsi-Hsin-Fu-Tzu-Tang 麻黃細辛附子湯*
(M.H. and Asarum Combination)
Main Herbs:
M.H. 4.0 grams, Asarum 3.0 grams, Aconite 1.0 grams.
Effects:
To be taken by those of delicate constitution with fever, severe chills, chilling of the limbs, and aching at the waist and back.
Uses:
Common cold, bronchitis, and bronchial asthma, in those of delicate constitution or the elderly.

81. Mai-Men-Tung-Tang 麥門冬湯 *
(Ophiopogon Combination)
Main Herbs:
Ophiopogon 10.0 grams, Pinellia 5.0 grams, Oryza 5.0 grams, Jujube 3.0 grams, Ginseng 2.0 grams, Licorice 2.0 grams.
Effects:
This formula is good to treat spasmodic cough due to congestion and characterized by the scanty sputum, dry mouth, hoarseness, and a feeling of dryness in the throat.
Uses:
Bronchitis, gasping, whooping cough, and hoarseness or loss of voice.

82. Sheng-Ling-Pai-Chu-San 參苓白朮散 ▲*
(Ginseng and Atractylodes Formula)

Main Herbs:
Ginseng 3.0 grams, Atractylodes 3.0 grams, Hoelen 3.0 grams, Licorice 1.5 grams, Dioscorea 1.5 grams, Dolichos 4.0 grams, Coix 5.0 grams, Lotus seeds 4.0 grams, Cardamon 2.0 grams, Platycodon 2.0 grams.
Effects:
This formula is good for the spleen and stomach. It is effective for those with gastrointestinal weakness, indigestion, vomiting or diarrhea, and loss of appetite.
Uses:
Chronic gastroenteritis, gastroptosis, chronic diarrhea, and fermentative indigestion.

83. Ching-Pi-Tang 清鼻湯
(Pueraria Nasal Combination)
Main Herbs:
Pueraria 4.0 grams, Cnidium 2.0 grams, M-4 4.0 grams, Rhubarb 1.0 gram, Cinnamon 2.0 grams, Licorice 1.0 gram, Paeonia 2.0 grams, Coix 3.0 grams, Platycodon 3.0 grams, Gypsum 2.0 grams, Magnolia flower 2.0 grams, Ginger 1.0 gram, Jujube 3.0 grams.
Effects:
This is the best known oral medication for the control of nasal discharge. It is effective for those who suffer from sinusitis, with heaviness in the head, emotional instability, loss of memory and retarded imagination.
Uses:
Nose suppuration, chronic rhinitis, and nasal congestion.

84. Ching-Sheng-Fang-Feng-Tang 清上防風湯 *
(Siler Combination)
Main Herbs:
Schizonepeta 1.5 grams, Coptis 1.5 grams, Mentha 1.5 grams, Chih-Shih 1.5 grams, Licorice 1.5 grams, Gardenia 3.0 grams, Cnidium 3.0 grams, Scute 3.0 grams, Forsythia 3.0 grams,

Angelica 3.0 grams, Platycodon 3.0 grams, Siler 3.0 grams.
Effects:
This formula is good to treat internal heat in the upper warmer and acne.
Uses:
Adolescent acne, eczema on the head, and red nose.

85. Ching-Fei-Tang 清肺湯 ▲ *
(Platycodon and Fritillary Combination)
Main Herbs:
Scute 2.0 grams, Platycodon 2.0 grams, Hoelen 3.0 grams, Citrus 2.0 grams, Tang-Kuei 3.0 grams, Morus 2.0 grams, Fritillary 2.0 grams, Ophiopogon 3.0 grams, Asparagus 2.0 grams, Almond 2.0 grams, Gardenia 2.0 grams, Schizandra 1.5 grams, Licorice 1.0 grams.
Effects:
This formula is good to treat coughing, especially when it is accompanied by internal heat in the lungs, and copious sputum.
Uses:
Bronchitis and bronchodilation.

86. Huang-Lien-Chiai-Tu-Tang 黃連解毒湯 *
(Coptis and Scute Combination)
Main Herbs:
Scute 3.0 grams, Coptis 2.0 grams, Phellodendron 2.0 grams, Gardenia 2.0 grams.
Effects:
This formula is effective for vertigo, stagnant blood, emotional instability, hemoptysis, nosebleed, and hemorrhoidal bleeding.
Uses:
Hemoptysis, uterine bleeding, nosebleeds, hypertension, and stomatitis.

87. Huang-Chi-Chien-Chung-Tang 黃耆建中湯 *
(Astragalus Combination)

Main Herbs:
Paeonia 6.0 grams, Cinnamon 3.0 grams, Ginger 3.0 grams, Jujube 3.0 grams, Licorice 3.0 grams, Astragalus 1.5 grams, Maltose 20 grams.

Effects:
This formula is good for suppuration occurring in those of chronic delicate constitution, or for convalescent symptoms.

Uses:
Weakness during convalescence, night sweats, otitis media, chronic ulcers, hemorrhoids, carbuncle, and children of delicate constitution.

88. Chu-Ling-Tang　豬苓湯　　　　　　　　　*
(Polyporus Combination)

Main Herbs:
Polyporus 3.0 grams, Hoelen 3.0 grams, Talcum 3.0 grams, Alisma 3.0 grams, Gelatin 3.0 grams.

Effects:
It is very effective for difficult or painful urination and hematuria.

Uses:
Nephritis, cystitis, urethritis, and urinary calculi (stones).

89. Hua-Kai-San　華蓋散　　　　　　　　　▲
(M.H. and Morus Formula)

Main Herbs:
M-4 4.0 grams, Almond 4.0 grams, Hoelen 5.0 grams, Citrus 2.0 grams, Morus 2.0 grams, Perilla fruit 2.0 grams, Licorice 1.0 grams.

Effects:
This formula is effective for cough with stridor and gastrointestinal weakness. It is especially good for children's cough with stridor.

Uses:
Common cold, bronchitis, bronchial asthma, and whooping cough.

90. Shu-Chin-Li-An-San 舒筋立安散
(Clematis and Carthamus Formula)
Main Herbs:
Siler 1.0 grams, Qianghuo 1.0 grams, Tuhuo 1.0 grams, Cnidium 1.0 grams, Hoelen 1.0 grams, Angelica 1.0 grams, Rehmannia 1.0 grams, Atractylodes 1.0 grams, Carthamus 1.0 grams, Persica 1.0 grams, Arisaema 1.0 grams, Citrus 1.0 grams, Pinellia 1.0 grams, Clematis 1.0 grams, Achyranthes 1.0 grams, Chaeonomelis 1.0 grams, Stephania 1.0 grams, Forsythia 1.0 grams, Scute 1.0 grams, Akebia 1.0 grams, Licorice 1.0 grams, Aconite 1.0 grams, Gentiana 1.0 grams, Bamboo sap 1.0 grams.
Effects:
This formula is good for chronic rheumatoid arthritis.
Uses:
Acute or chronic rheumatoid arthritis, rheumatic pain in the knees, and hemiplegia.

91. Shu-Ching-Huo-hsieh-Tang 疏經活血湯 *
(Clematis and Stephania Combination)
Main Herbs:
Paeonia 2.5 grams, Tang-Kuei 2.0 grams, Cnidium 2.0 grams, Rehmannia 2.0 grams, Atractylodes 2.0 grams, Persica 2.0 grams, Hoelen 2.0 grams, Achyranthes 1.5 grams, Clematis 1.5 grams, Stephania 1.5 grams, Qianghuo 1.5 grams, Siler 1.5 grams, Gentiana 1.5 grams, Angelica 1.0 grams, Citrus 1.5 grams, Licorice 1.0 grams, Ginger 1.5 grams.
Effects:
This formula is good for those of delicate constitution due to excessive drinking or sexual life. It is also good for migratory aches which are especially severe in the left leg during the night.
Uses:
Neuralgia, sciatica, and muscular rheumatism.

92. Yueh-Pi-Chia-Chu-Tang 越婢加朮湯
(Atractylodes Combination)

Main Herbs:
M.H. 6.0 grams, Gypsum 8.0 grams, Ginger 3.0 grams, Licorice 2.0 grams, Jujube 3.0 grams, Atractylodes 4.0 grams.
Effects:
It is good for edema or sweats, difficulty in urination, skin diseases, urological diseases, eye ailments, and rheumatism.
Uses:
Acute nephritis, edema of nephritis, rheumatoid arthritis, eczema, and acute conjuctivitis.

93. Kou-Teng-San 鈞藤散 *
(Gambir Formula)
Main Herbs:
Gambir 3.0 grams, Citrus 3.0 grams, Pinellia 3.0 grams, Ophiopogen 3.0 grams, Hoelen 3.0 grams, Ginger 1.0 grams, Gypsum 5.0 grams, Ginseng 2.0 grams, Chrysanthemum 2.0 grams, Siler 2.0 grams, Licorice 1.0 grams.
Effects:
This formula is frequently used for nervous symptoms after middle age such as headache, vertigo, shoulder stiffness, hypertension, and arteriosclerosis.
Uses:
Headache due to cerebral arteriosclerosis, or of emotional origin, and insomnia.

94. Wen-Ching-Tang 溫經湯 ▲*
(Tang-Kuei and Evodia Combination)
Main Herbs:
Evodia 1.0 grams, Tang-Kuei 3.0 grams, Cnidium 2.0 grams, Ginseng 2.0 grams, Cinnamon 2.0 grams, Gelatin 2.0 grams, Moutan 2.0 grams, Ginger 1.0 grams, Paeonia 2.0 grams, Licorice 2.0 grams, Pinellia 5.0 grams, Ophiopogon 5.0 grams.
Effects:
This formula is good for treatment of women with a chill

86

constitution, hot palms, dry lips, and menstrual irregularities.
Uses:
Menstrual irregularities, infertility, menopausal disorders,
leucorrhea, eczema, and thickening and hardening of the skin
on the palm of the hand.

95. Wen-Ching-Yin 溫清飲 *

(Tang-Kuei and Gardenia Combination)
Main Herbs:
Tang-Kuei 4.0 grams, Rehmannia 4.0 grams, Paeonia 4.0
grams, Cnidium 4.0 grams, Coptis 1.5 grams, Scute 3.0
grams, Phellodendron 1.5 grams, Gardenia 2.0 grams.
Effects:
This is a combined formula of Szu-Wu-Tang (Tang-Kuei Four
Combination) and Huang-Lien-Chiai-Tu-Tang (Coptis and
Scute Combination). It is effective for skin diseases and
eczema in those of the anemic constitution.
Uses:
Bleeding, uterine bleeding, anemia, eczema, dermatitis, and
freckles.

96. Pu-Chung-I-Chi-Tang 補中益氣湯 ▲ *

(Ginseng and Astragalus Combination)
Main Herbs:
Astragalus 4.0 grams, Ginseng 4.0 grams, Licorice 1.5 grams,
Atractylodes 4.0 grams, Citrus 2.0 grams, Tang-Kuei 3.0
grams, Cimicifuga 1.0 grams, Bupleurum 2.0 grams, Ginger
2.0 grams, Jujube 2.0 grams.
Effects:
This is a famous tonic formula for those having a tendency
towards anemia, fatigue, and loss of appetite. It is also
effective in preventing weight loss during the summer.
Uses:
Convalescent weakness, anemia, delicate constitution,
hemorrhoids, prolapse of the rectum, and susceptibility to
indigestion.

97. Tzu-Sheng-Ming-Mu-Tang 滋腎明目湯 ▲
(Chrysanthemum Combination)
Main Herbs:
Tang-Kuei 3.0 grams, Paeonia 3.0 grams, Cnidium 3.0 grams, Rehmannia 6.0 grams, Platycodon 1.5 grams, Ginseng 1.5 grams, Gardenia 1.5 grams, Coptis 1.5 grams, Angelica 1.5 grams, Vitex 1.5 grams, Chrysanthemum 1.5 grams, Licorice 1.5 grams, Juncus 1.5 grams, Tea 1.5 grams.
Effects:
This formula is good for visual disturbances and cataract due to lingering disease or delicate constitution.
Uses:
Visual disturbance, eye fatigue, and cataract.

98. Tzu-Sheng-Tung-Erh-Tang 滋腎通耳湯 ▲
(Scute Combination)
Main Herbs:
Tang-Kuei 3.0 grams, Cnidium 3.0 grams, Paeonia 3.0 grams, Anemmarrhena 3.0 grams, Rehmannia 3.0 grams, Phellodendron 3.0 grams, Scute 3.0 grams, Burpleurum 3.0 grams, Angelica 3.0 grams, Cyperus 3.0 grams.
Effects:
This formula is effective for tinnitus and difficulty in hearing due to kidney weakness.
Uses:
Hearing loss due to otitis media, old age, and drug side-effects.

99. Tang-Kuei-Shao-Yao-San 當歸芍藥散 *
(Tang-Kuei and Peony Formula)
Main Herbs:
Tang-Kuei 3.0 grams, Cnidium 3.0 grams, Paeonia 4.0 grams, Hoelen 4.0 grams, Atractylodes 4.0 grams, Alisma 4.0 grams.
Effects:
This has been a very popular formula for female disorders. It

is effective for improving the blood circulation, and as a body tonic for women with chills. It is also a good preventive for miscarriage.

Uses:

Menstrual irregularities, anemia before or after childbirth, nephritis, black spots on the skin, habitual abortion, and hemorrhoids.

100. Tang-Kuei-Szu-Ni-Chia-Wu-Chu-Yu-Shen-Chiang-Tang 當歸四逆加吳茱萸生薑湯 *

(Tang Kuei and Evodia and Ginger Combination)

Main Herbs:

Tang-Kuei 3.0 grams, Cinnamon 3.0 grams, Paeonia 3.0 grams, Asarum 2.0 grams, Licorice 2.0 grams, Akebia 3.0 grams, Jujube 5.0 grams, Evodia 2.0 grams, Ginger 4.0 grams.

Effects:

This formula is good for chills or chronic pain. It is also good for preventing chilblain and for improving blood circulation.

Uses:

Frigorism, neuralgia, dysmenorrhea, and abdominal pain originating in the uterus.

101. Ko-Ken-Tang 葛根湯 *

(Pueraria Combination)

Main Herbs:

Pueraria 8.0 grams, M.H. 4.0 grams, Cinnamon 3.0 grams, Licorice 2.0 grams, Paeonia 3.0 grams, Ginger 1.0 gram, Jujube 4.0 grams.

Effects:

This formula is good for a common cold without perspiration but with severe chills, stiffness of the neck and back, and inflammation.

Uses:

Common cold, suppuration, neuralgia, eczema, acute colitis, furuncle, boils, and tonsillitis.

102. Ko-Ken-Huang-Lien-Huang-Chin-Tang   *
(Pueraria, Coptis and Scute Combination) 葛根黃連黃芩湯
Main Herbs:
Pueraria 6.0 grams, Coptis 3.0 grams, Scute 3.0 grams, Licorice 2.0 grams.
Effects:
To be taken by those having diarrhea, fever associated with shoulder stiffness, and vomiting due to drunkenness.
Uses:
Acute gastroenteritis, colitis, diarrhea, drunkenness, hypertension, and "stomach flu."

103. Suan-Tsao-Jen-Tang 酸棗仁湯   *
(Zizyphus Combination)
Main Herbs:
Zizyphus 1.5 grams, Hoelen 5.0 grams, Anemarrhena 3.0 grams, Cnidium 3.0 grams, Licorice 1.0 gram.
Effects:
It is effective for insomnia in those of delicate constitution or because of fatigue.
Uses:
Insomnia, night sweats, and amnesia.

104. Lo-Shih-Shu 樂適舒
(W.T.T.C.)
Main Herbs:
Coix 8.0 grams, Terminalia 8.0 grams, Trapa 8.0 grams, Wistaria 8.0 grams.
Effects:
Forty percent cure rate of stomach cancer and rectal carcinoma, inhibition of multiplication of cancer cells, and prevention of metastases of the postoperative cancer.
Uses:
Inflammation, difficulty in urination, edema, arthritis, pain, and convulsions.

105. Lung-Tan-Hsieh-Kan-Tang 龍膽瀉肝湯 ▲ *
(Gentiana Combination)
Main Herbs:
Tang-Kuei 5.0 grams, Rehmannia 5.0 grams, Scute 3.0 grams, Gardenia 1.0 grams, Akebia 5.0 grams, Plantago 3.0 grams, Licorice 1.0 grams, Gentiana 1.0 grams, Alisma 3.0 grams.
Effects:
This formula is good to treat fever, inflammation, blood fever, and dysuria. It is effective for inflammation in the lower abdomen and genital areas, and for congestion, swelling, and pain.
Uses:
Cystitis, urethritis, vaginitis, leucorrhea, endometritis, genital pruritis, and gonorrhea.

106. I-Yi-Jen-Tang 薏苡仁湯 *
(Coix Combination)
Main Herbs:
Tang-Kuei 4.0 grams, Coix 8.0 grams, Atractylodes 4.0 grams, Paeonia 3.0 grams, Cinnamon 3.0 grams, M.H. 4.0 grams, Licorice 2.0 grams.
Effects:
It is very effective for subclinical arthritis and rheumatism with pain, swelling, and fever.
Uses:
Rheumatoid arthritis, muscular rheumatism, and osteoarthritis.

107. Kuei-Pi-Tang 歸脾湯 *
(Ginseng and Longan Combination)
Main Herbs:
Ginseng 3.0 grams, Astragalus 2.0 grams, Longan 3.0 grams, Atractylodes 3.0 grams, Hoelen 3.0 grams, Ginger 1.0 grams, Tang-Kuei 2.0 grams, Jujube 1.0 grams, Polygala 1.0 grams, Inula 1.0 grams, Licorice 1.0 grams, Zizyphus 3.0 grams.

Effects:
This formula is good for those of delicate constitution with gastrointestinal weakness; also for bleeding, anemia, amnesia, and neurosis brought on by physical and mental overwork.
Uses:
Nervous exhaustion, insomnia, amnesia, anemia, menstrual irregularities, and loss of appetite due to bleeding.

108. Hsiang-Sheng-Po-Ti-Wan 響聲破笛丸   *
(Gasping Formula)
Main Herbs:
Forsythia 2.5 grams, Platycodon 2.5 grams, Licorice 2.5 grams, Rhubarb 1.0 grams, Cardamon 1.0 grams, Cnidium 1.0 grams, Myrobalans 1.0 grams, Catechu 2.0 grams, Mentha 4.0 grams.
Effects:
This formula is good to treat hoarseness due to excessive speaking and singing.
Uses:
Hoarseness and sore throat.

109. Hsu-Ming-Tang 續命湯
(Ma Huang and Ginseng Combination)
Main Herbs:
Almond 4.0 grams, Ma Huang 3.0 grams, Cinnamon 3.0 grams, Ginseng 3.0 grams, Tang-Kuei 3.0 grams, Cnidium 2.0 grams, Ginger 2.0 grams, Licorice 2.0 grams, Gypsum 6.0 grams.
Effects:
This formula is good for hemiplegia or speaking difficulty due to stroke, and accompanied by headache, stridor, and thirst.
Uses:
Motor or language difficulty, hypertension, cerebromalacia, and moneplegia after stroke.

110. Pien-Chih-Hsin-Chi-Yin 變製心氣飲
(Areca and Evodia Combination)

Main Herbs:
Cinnamon 2.5 grams, Areca Seed 2.5 grams, Hoelen 5.0 grams, Pinellia 5.0 grams, Akebia 2.5 grams, Perilla fruit 2.0 grams, Tortoise shell 2.0 grams, Chih-Shih 2.0 grams, Morus 1.0 grams, Licorice 1.0 grams, Evodia 1.0 grams.
Effects:
It is good for palpitations, rapid respiration, edema, stiffness of the shoulders and back, and cardiac asthma.
Uses:
Cardiac asthma, chronic bronchitis, and angina pectoris.

111. Chi-Li-San 七厘散 ▲
(Musk and Catechu Formula)
Main Herbs:
Carthamus 0.8 grams, Cinnabar 0.5 grams, Calamus gum 4.0 grams, Musk 0.05 grams, Borneol 0.05 grams, Mastic 0.6 grams, Myrrh 0.8 grams, Catechu 1.0 grams.
Uses:
External injuries, stagnant blood, and generalized body aches.

112. Li-Ke-Tang 利膈湯
(Pinellia and Gardenia Combination)
Main Herbs:
Pinellia 3.0 grams, Aconite 1.0 grams, Gardenia 3.0 grams.
Effects:
This formula is effective for a sensation of constriction in the throat, difficulty in swallowing, vomiting, viscid sputum, and thirst.
Uses:
Esophageal constriction, spasm due to carcinoma, and gastric cancer.

113. Hsin-I-San 辛夷散
(Magnolia Flower Formula)

Main Herbs:
Magnolia flower 1.5 grams, Angelica 2.5 grams, Cimicifuga 1.0 grams, Ko-pun 1.5 grams, Qianghuo 2.5 grams, Siler 2.5 grams, Cnidium 2.5 grams, Asarum 1.5 grams, Akebia 2.5 grams, Licorice 1.0 grams.
Effects:
This formula is good to treat the symptoms of nasal congestion and continuous postnasal drainage. It is also effective for nasal congestion and headache due to a common cold.
Uses:
Coryza and chronic rhinitis.

114. Chai-Ling-Tang 柴苓湯 *
(Bupleurum and Hoelen Combination)
Main Herbs:
Bupleurum 5.0 grams, Pinellia 4.0 grams, Ginger 4.0 grams, Scute 2.5 grams, Jujube 2.5 grams, Ginseng 2.5 grams, Licorice 2.0 grams, Alisma 4.0 grams, Polyporus 2.5 grams, Atractylodes, 2.5 grams, Hoelen 2.5 grams, Cinnamon 2.5 grams.
Effects:
This is a combined formula consisting of Hsiao-Chai-Hu-Tang (Minor Bupleurum Combination) and Wu-Ling-San (Hoelen Five Herbs Formula). It is good for thirst, edema, diarrhea, or difficult micturition.
Uses:
Common cold, acute gastroenteritis, nephritis, and pyelitis.

115. Chai-Hsien-Tang 柴陷湯
(Bupleurum and Scute Combination)
Main Herbs:
Bupleurum 5.0 grams, Pinellia 5.0 grams, Scute 3.0 grams, Ginseng 2.0 grams, Jujube 3.0 grams, Ginger 3.0 grams, Licorice 1.5 grams, Coptis 1.5 grams, Trichosanthes Seed 3.0 grams.

Effects:
This is a combination formula consisting of Hsiao-Chai-Hu-Tang (Minor Bupleurum Combination) with Coptis and Trichosanthes Seed. It is to be taken for pain in the chest during coughing or deep breathing, for a feeling of fullness and pressure in the chest, and for dry mouth, rapid respirations, viscid sputum, and lingering chills and fever.
Uses:
Bronchitis, pneumonia, pleuritis, and the common cold.

116. Kuei-Chih-Shao-Yao-Chih-Mu-Tang 桂枝芍藥知母湯
(Cinnamon and Anemarrhena Combination)
Main Herbs:
Cinnamon 3.0 grams, Anemarrhena 3.0 grams, Siler 3.0 grams, Ginger 3.0 grams, Paeonia 3.0 grams, M.H. 3.0 grams, Atractylodes 4.0 grams, Licorice 1.5 grams, Aconite 1.0 grams.
Effects:
This formula is good for treatment of chronic arthropathy in those of delicate constitution.
Use:
Chronic arthritis.

117. Sang-Chu-Yin 桑菊飲 ▲
(Morus and Chrysanthemum Combination)
Main Herbs:
Morus leaves 6.0 grams, Chrysanthemum 2.0 grams, Almond 4.0 grams, Forsythia 3.0 grams, Mentha 2.0 grams, Platycodon 4.0 grams, Licorice 2.0 grams, Phragmites 4.0 grams.
Effects:
This formula is suitable for the early stages of leprosy, fever, cough, and mild thirst.
Uses:
Common cold, headache, vertigo, fever, and cough.

118. Ching-Liang-Yin 清涼飲
(Gardenia and Mentha Combination)
Main Herbs:
Gardenia 2.5 grams, Forsythia 2.5 grams, Siler 2.5 grams, Scute 2.0 grams, Chih-Ko 2.5 grams, Tang-Kuei 2.0 grams, Ginger 2.0 grams, Platycodon 2.0 grams, Coptis 1.0 grams, Licorice 1.0 grams, Mentha 1.0 grams, Rehmannia 2.0 grams.
Effects:
This formula is good for the treatment of internal heat and pain due to swelling in the throat.
Uses:
Tonsillitis, and pain due to swelling in the throat.

119. Ching-Wei-San 清胃散
(Coptis and Rehmannia Formula)
Main Herbs:
Gypsum 10.0 grams, Moutan 4.0 grams, Scute 2.5 grams, Rehmannia 2.5 grams, Coptis 2.5 grams, Cimicifuga 2.5 grams.
Effects:
This formula is effective in the treatment of pyorrhea, bleeding of the dental pulp, and febrile stomach.
Uses:
Stomatitis, pain due to swelling in the throat, and toothache.

120. Tzu-Yun-Kao 紫雲膏 *
(Lithospermum Ointment)
Main Herbs:
Sesame oil 1000 grams, Tang-Kuei 100 grams, Lithospermum 100 grams, Flava wax 380 grams, Lard 25 grams.
Effects:
This ointment is used mainly for inflammation, bleeding, bacterial infection, pain, physical weakness, and granulation. It is also effective for cracks on the hands and feet, ulcers, abnormal multiplicaion of skin tissue, suppuration, and itching of skin lesions.

Uses:
Burns, cracks on the hands and feet, chilblain, lesions, hemorrhoids, and inflammation.

121. Tzu-Yin-Chiang-Ho-Tang　滋陰降火湯　　　*
(Phellodendron Combination)
Main Herbs:
Tang-Kuei 2.5 grams, Paeonia 2.5 grams, Rehmannia 2.5 grams, Asparagus 2.5 grams, Ophiopogon 2.5 grams, Citrus 2.5 grams, Atractylodes 3.0 grams, Anemarrhena 1.5 grams, Phellodendron 1.5 grams, Licorice 1.5 grams.
Effects:
This formula is recommended for thirst, insomnia, rapid respirations, hyperplastic tuberculosis, and for regulating body fluids.
Uses:
Tuberculosis, pleurisy without expectoration, bronchitis, pyelitis, and diabetes.

122. Wen-Tan-Tang　溫膽湯　　　*
(Bamboo and Hoelen Combination)
Main Herbs:
Pinellia 6.0 grams, Hoelen 6.0 grams, Ginger 3.0 grams, Citrus 2.5 grams, Bamboo 2.0 grams, Licorice 1.0 grams, Chih-Shih 1.5 grams.
Effects:
This formula is to be taken by those of atonic constitution who have insomnia due to gastroptosis or atonic stomach.
Uses:
Insomnia, anxiety, palpitations, and gastrointestinal disturbances.

葛根湯加川芎、辛夷

123. Ko-Ken-Tang-Chia-Chuan-Chiung-Hsin-I　　　*
(Pueraria and Magnolia Combination)

Main Herbs:
Pueraria 4.0 grams, M-4 4.0 grams, Cinnamon 2.0 grams, Licorice 2.0 grams, Paeonia 2.0 grams, Ginger 1.0 grams, Cnidium 3.0 grams, Magnolia 3.0 grams, Jujube 3.0 grams.
Uses:
Coryza, chronic rhinitis, and nasal congestion.

124. Tsang-Erh-San 蒼耳散
(Xanthium Formula)
Main Herbs:
Angelica 3.0 grams, Mentha 3.0 grams, Magnolia flower 3.0 grams, Xanthium 5.0 grams.
Uses:
Coryza and chronic rhinitis.

125. Pu-Kung-Ying-Tang 蒲公英湯
(Dandelion Combination)
Main Herbs:
Dandelion 8.0 grams, Tang-Kuei 6.0 grams, Dioscorea 4.0 grams, Cyperus 3.0 grams, Moutan 3.0 grams.
Effects:
This formula is recommended for treatment of agalactia; it should be taken within one month after childbirth.
Uses:
As a lactagogue.

126. Teng-Hua-Pai-Tu-San 燈花敗毒散
(Ludwigia Formula)
Main Herbs:
Ludwigia 6.0 grams, Hoelen 3.0 grams, Rhubarb 1.2 grams, Lithospermum 3.0 grams, Polygonum 3.6 grams, Polyporus 3.0 grams, Alisma 3.0 grams, Gleditschia spine 3.6 grams, Ginger 0.6 grams.
Effects:

This formula is recommended for toxemia, inflammation, and polyuria. It is especially effective for primary urticaria.
Uses:
Urticaria and pruritis.

127. Tu-Huo-Chi-Shen-Tang　獨活寄生湯　　▲＊
(Tu-huo and Viscum Combination)
Main Herbs:
Tuhuo 3.0 grams, Vaeicum 2.0 grams, Chin-Chiu 2.0 grams, Siler 2.0 grams, Asarum 2.0 grams, Tang-Kuei 2.0 grams, Paeonia 2.0 grams, Cnidium 2.0 grams, Rehmannia 2.0 grams, Eucommia 2.0 grams, Achyranthes 2.0 grams, Ginseng 2.0 grams, Hoelen 2.0 grams, Licorice 2.0 grams, Cinnamon 2.0 grams.
Effects:
This formula can regulate blood circulation and is effective as an analgesic and antispasmodic. It is good for rheumatism and osteoarthritis in those of weak confirmation and for pain in the chest and back during pregnancy. It is not effective for acute rheumatic conditions.
Uses:
Lumbago, pain or numbness in the knees and feet, neuralgia, and rheumatism.

128. Huan-Shao-Tan　還少丹　　　　　　▲
(Lycium Formula)
Main Herbs:
Anemone 1.2 grams, Dioscorea 1.2 grams, Achyranthes 1.2 grams, Cornus 1.2 grams, Polygala 1.2 grams, Morinda 1.2 grams, Schizandra 1.2 grams, Cistanche 1.2 grams, Broussonetia 1.2 grams, Hoelen 1.2 grams, Lycium 1.2 grams, Rehmannia 1.2 grams, Fennel 1.2 grams, Eucommia 1.2 grams, Jujube 3.6 grams.
Effects:
This is a tonic formula for stimulating proper functioning of

the heart, kidneys, spleen, and stomach. It is effective in the treatment of anorexia, fever, night sweats, toothache, pain at the waist, fatigue, uterine diseases, and abnormal emission. It also increases vigor.

Uses:

Weakness and decrease of libido.

PART III

Some Commonly Used Chinese Herbs

CHINESE HERBS

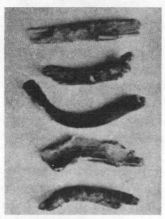

Acanthopanax

ACANTHOPANACIS CORTEX
五加皮

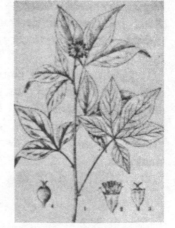

Chinese Name: (Wu-Chia-Pi)

Acanthopanacis Cortex is a superior drug recorded in *The Herbal by Shen Nung* (A.D. 25-220). Botanically, it is the epidermis of the dried root of the 2 to 3 meter tall, deciduous shrub, *Acanthopanax gracilistylus* W. W. Smith of the Araliaceae family.

Its chemical components are 4-Methoxysalicyl aldehyde, Vitamin A, and b-sitosterol. It is used as a nutritive tonic and aphrodaisiac. Chinese medicine gives it for impotence, itching due to moisture near the scrotum, muscle spasms due to rheumatism, and convulsions.

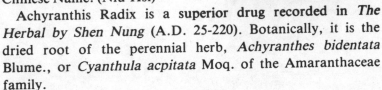

Achyranthes

ACHYRANTHIS RADIX
牛膝

Chinese Name: (Niu-Hsi)

Achyranthis Radix is a superior drug recorded in *The Herbal by Shen Nung* (A.D. 25-220). Botanically, it is the dried root of the perennial herb, *Achyranthes bidentata* Blume., or *Cyanthula acpitata* Moq. of the Amaranthaceae family.

It is a diuretic and emmenagogue, and Chinese medicine uses it for amenorrhea, gonorrhea, hematuria, swelling carbuncles, dystocia, and for dispelling stagnant blood. The brewed root is used for treating weakness of the liver and kidneys, pain in the waist and knees, and generalized weakness.

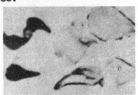

Aconite

ACONITI RADIX (WOLF'S BANE)
附子

Chinese Name: (Fu-Tzu)

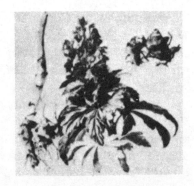

Aconiti Radix is the affiliated tuberous root of *Aconitum carmichaeli* Debx. of the Ranunculaceae family. Because it is like a son affiliated to the mother, it is named Fu (affiliated) Tzu (son). This plant is recorded in the earliest Chinese herb classic, *The Herbal by Shen Nung,* and has a number of species. Aconite or Wolf's Bane *(Aconitum napellus)* and this plant are in the same genus.

Since ancient times, Chinese have processed Aconiti Radix in order to decrease its toxicities for safe administration, i.e., to transform the main component Aconitin to Benzoyl Aconin. Western medicine uses it for neuralgia, while Chinese medicine uses it for weak constitution, poor metabolism, dysuria, cardiac weakness, gout, rheumatism in the limbs, neuralgia, and chills.

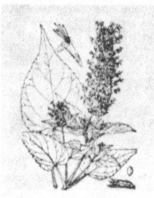

Agastache

AGASTACHIS
HERBA
藿香

Chinese Name: (Huo-Shiang)

Agastachis Herba is a commonly used drug first recorded in *Chia Yeou Pen Tsao* (A.D. 1061). Botanically, it is the dried, whole plant of the annual herb, *Agastache rugosa* (Fisch. et Mey.) O. Kuntze. of the Labiatae family.

It is used as an aromatic stomachic, refrigerant, and antipyretic. It is effective for dyspepsia, vomiting with diarrhea, abdominal pain, chest distension due to gastric disorders, the common cold, and headache.

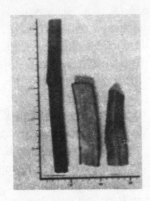

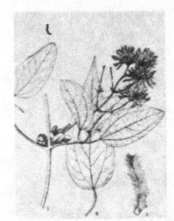

Akebia

AKEBIAE CAULIS
木通
Chinese Name: (Mu-Tung)

Akebiae Caulis, a general drug recorded in *The Herbal by Shen Nung,* is a stem with a small hollow in the center. Botanically, it is the dried stem of *Akebia quinata Decne* (Lardizabalaceae family) in Japan and of *Clematis armandi* (Ranunculaceae family) in China. Since the whole plant is a rattan resembling a shrub and the herb drug is hollow at both ends, it is called Mu (shrub) Tung (through).

Chinese medicine often uses Akebiae Caulis as a diuretic for edema, urethritis, nephritis, and cystitis. Its principal chemical constituents are Akebin, Hederagenin, and Oleanalic acid.

104

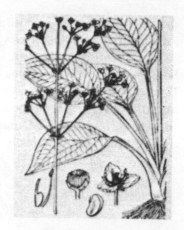

Alisma

ALISMATIS RHIZOMA (WATER PLANTAIN)

澤瀉

Chinese Name: (Tse-Hsieh)

Alismatis Rhizoma, a superior herb drug recorded in *The Herbal by Shen Nung,* is the dried subterranean root-like stem of the perennial *Alisma plantago-aquatica* L. var. *orientalis* of the Alismataceae family. It is most often grown in the swamp and the paddy field. Having a resemblance to Plantain, it possesses the scientific name *Plantago aquatica.*

Chinese medicine uses Alismatis Rhizoma for dysuria, thirst, and swelling of the lower abdomen.

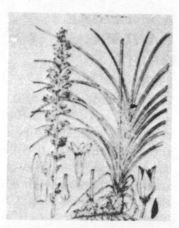

Anemarrhena

ANEMARRHENAE RHIZOMA

知母

Chinese Name: (Chih-Mu)

Anemarrhenae Rhizoma is a general drug first recorded in *The Herbal by Shen Nung* (A.D. 25-220). Botanically, it is the dried, subterranean, root-like stem of the perennial herb *Anemarrhena asphodeloides* Bunge of the Liliaceae family.

Its chemical components are Saponin, Asphonin, Sarsapogenin, Maykogenin, Neogitogenin, and Timosaponin. Because of its nutritive, tonic, anti-inflammative, sedative, and diuretic effects, Chinese medicine uses it for anxiety due to stress, fever, thirst, internal heat in the lungs, cough, debilitating fever, dry stools, and dysuria.

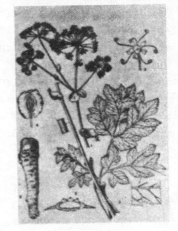

Angelica

ANGELICAE DAHURICAE RADIX

白芷

Chinese Name: (Pai-Chih)

Angelicae Dahuricae Radix was first recorded as a "drug" in one of the oldest Chinese books, *The Classic on Mountains and Seas* (B.C. 400). It is the root of *Angelica dahurica* or *A. dahurica* var. *pai-chi* of the Umbelliferae family. It is an annual wild-grown herb with a height of five inches or more and a root longer than a foot. The plant is white (Pai) and fragrant (Chih).

This herb drug may be used for the common cold, migraine, dizziness, neuralgia, and perspiration.

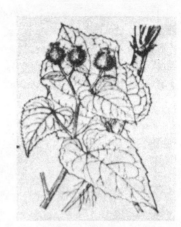

Arctium

ARCTII FRUCTUS
牛蒡子

Chinese Name: (Niu-Pang-Tzu)

Arctii Fructus is a general drug first recorded in *Ming I Pieh Lu* (A.D. 500). Botanically, it is the dried, ripe fruit of the biennial herb, 1 to 1.5 meter tall *Arctium lappa* L. of the Compositae family.

Its chemical components are arctiin and fatty oil. It has antitoxic, antipyretic, diuretic, and diaphoretic actions. Chinese medicine uses it for the common cold, cough, swelling and pain in the throat, swelling carbuncles, and measles.

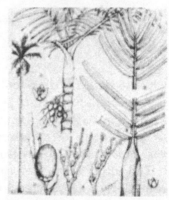

Areca Seed

ARECAE SEMEN
檳榔子

Chinese Name: (Pin-Lang Tzu)

Arecae Semen is a general drug recorded in *Ming I Pieh Lu* (A.D. 500). Botanically, it is the dried, ripe seed of the 10 to 18 meter tall *Areca catechu* L. of the Palmae family.

Its chemical components are Arecoline, Arecoidine, and Tannin. It is effective as a vermifuge, diuretic, and myotic. Chinese medicine uses it for malaria, abdominal distension and pain, evacuation of the uterus, and to promote gastrointestinal evacuation.

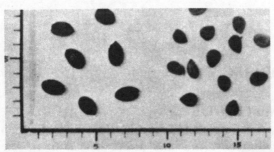

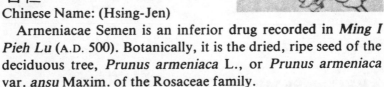

Apricot Seed (Almond)

ARMENIACAE
SEMEN
杏仁

Chinese Name: (Hsing-Jen)

Armeniacae Semen is an inferior drug recorded in *Ming I Pieh Lu* (A.D. 500). Botanically, it is the dried, ripe seed of the deciduous tree, *Prunus armeniaca* L., or *Prunus armeniaca* var. *ansu* Maxim. of the Rosaceae family.

The bitter kernels of the fruit are officinal. Its chemical components are amygdalin and emulsin. It is used as an expectorant, antitussive, and sedative. Chinese medicine uses it for coughing, wheezing, chest distension, spasms in the throat, and constipation.

Asarum

ASARI CUM RADICE HERBA

細辛

(WILD GINGER)

Chinese Name: (Hsi-Hsin)

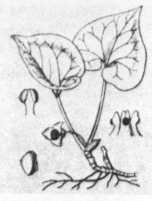

Asari Cum Radice Herba, first recorded in *The Herbal by Shen Nung,* is the slender root and root-like stem of the perennial *Asarum sieboldi* of the Aristolochiaceae family. Being slender and acrid, it is called Hsi (slender) Hsin (acrid).

This herb material may be used as a diaphoretic, expectorant, headache remedy, and diuretic. It is especially effective for stagnant water in the stomach, constant coughs, and chest distention.

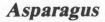

Asparagus

ASPARAGI RADIX

天門冬

Chinese Name: (Ten-Men-Tong)

Asparagi Radix is a superior drug recorded in *The Herbal by Shen Nung* (A.D. 25-220). Botanically, it is the dried bulb root of the creeping, perennial herb, *Asparagus cochinchinensis* (Loureiro) Merrill of the Liliaceae family.

The chemical components of this root are Asparagine and a viscous liquid which act together as a nutritive tonic, antipyretic, expectorant, antitussive, and diuretic. It is effective for coughing, dysuria, gout, heart disorders, and dropsy.

Astragalus

ASTRAGALI RADIX (YELLOW VETCH)

黃耆

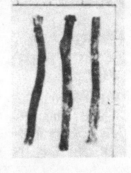

Chinese Name: (Huang-Chi)

Astragali Radix is a superior drug in *The Herbal by Shen Nung* and is called "the superior tonic" in *Pen Tsao Kang Mu* (The General Catalog of Herbs). Botanically, it is the dried root of the perennial *Astragalus membranaceus* (Fischer) Bunge or *A. mongholicus Bunge* of the Leguminosae family *(Hedysarum sp.)*.

This herb is used for general weakness, malnutrition, night sweats, anascara, difficulty in urination, and diarrhea.

Atractylodes

ATRACTYLODIS ALBA RHIZOMA

白术

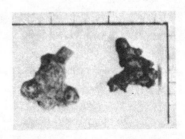

(ATRACTYLODES; CHU)

Chinese Name: (Pai-Chu)

Atractylodis Alba Rhizoma, a superior drug recorded in *The Herbal by Shen Nung,* has been commonly used in Chinese medicine. Botanically, it is the dried subterranean root-like stem of the wild perennial two to three-foot herb, *Atractylodes macrocephala Koidz* of the Compositae family.

110

This is a very important herb drug used mainly for polyuria or dysuria, stagnant water in the stomach, dizziness, watery diarrhea, and as an aromatic stomachic for edema, night sweats, vomiting in pregnancy, and unstable fetus. It contains an essential oil (3.5 to 6.0%) and the main component atractylone.

Ts'ang-Chu are the dried subterranean root-like stems of the same genera, *A. lancea* and *A. chinensis*. Being good for the spleen and in dispersing moisture, they are used for vomiting and diarrhea, visceral swelling, and related disturbances.

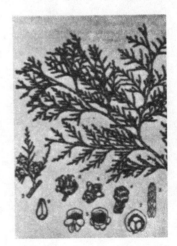

Biota

BIOTAE SEMEN
柏子仁

Chinese Name: (Po-Tzu-Jen)

Biotae Semen is a superior drug recorded in *The Herbal by Shen Nung* (A.D. 25-220). Botanically, it is the dried, ripe seed of the 10 to 15 meter tall, evergreen tree, *Biota orientalis* (L.) Endl. of the Cupressaceae family.

It is a nutritive tonic, expectorant, and antitussive agent. Chinese medicine uses it for palpitations, insomnia, amnesia, delicate constitution, ephidrosis, spermatorrhea, constipation, congestion, bronchitis, asthma, and dry stools.

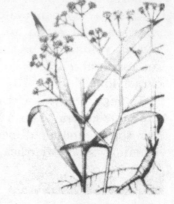

Bupleurum

BUPLEURI RADIX
(HARE'S EAR)

柴胡

Chinese Name: (Chai-Hu)

Bupleuri Radix, a superior herb drug recorded in *The Herbal by Shen Nung,* has been commonly used in Chinese medicine. Botanically, it is the dried root of *Bupleurum chinensis* or *B. scorzoneraefolium* of the Umbelliferae family.

Bupleuri Radix has antipyretic, antitoxic, analgesic, sedative, and antitussive properties. Chinese medicine uses it for chest distress and congestion, alternating chill and fever, and respiratory ailments. It is also used to improve liver function. Professor Shibata of Tokyo University isolated from it a saponin named saikogenin which has been proven anti-edematous by Professor Takagi of the same university.

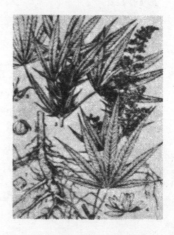

Cannabis Seed

CANNABIS SEMEN

大麻仁

Chinese Name: (Ta-Ma-Jen)

Cannabis Semen is a superior drug first recorded in *The Herbal by Shen Nung* (A.D. 25-220). Botanically, it is the dried ripe seeds of the annual, one to three meter tall herb, *Cannabis sativa* L. of the Cannabinaceae family.

Chinese medicine considers these seeds to be a nutritive tonic with vermifugal and emollient properties; they are used for constipation and internal heat in the intestines. The alkaloid in the leaves is not present in the seeds.

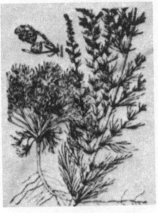

Capillaris

ARTEMISIAE CAPILLARIS HERBA
茵陳

Chinese Name: (Yin-Chen)

Artemisiae Capillaris Herba is a superior drug recorded in *The Herbal by Shen Nung* (A.D. 25-220). Botanically, it is the dried whole plant of the perennial herb, *Artemisia capillaris* Thunb. of the Compositae family, which grows in gravelly river banks.

Its chemical components are b-pinene and capillene which have been shown to have vermifugal, diuretic, and anti-inflammative effects. Chinese medicine uses it for jaundice, difficulty in urination, and skin diseases.

113

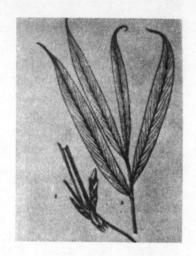

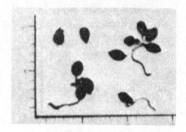

Cardamon

AMOMI FRUCTUS
seu SEMEN
砂仁

Chinese Name: (Sha-Jen)

Amomi Fructus seu Semen is a commonly used drug first recorded in *Kai Pao Pen Tsao* (A.D. 973). Botanically, it is the dried, ripe seed or fruit of the perennial herb, *Amomum villosum* Lour., or *Amomum xanthioides* Wall., of Zingiberaceae family.

Chinese medicine recognizes its aromatic and stomachic effects and uses it for treating abdominal distention, stagnant food in the stomach, gastric disorders, vomiting, diarrhea, and for suppressing uterine contractions during pregnancy.

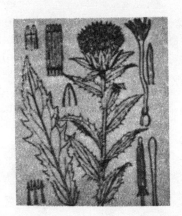

Carthamus

CARTHAMI FLOS
紅花
Chinese Name: (Hung-Hua)

Carthami Flos is a commonly used drug first recorded in *Kai Pao Pen Tsao* (A.D. 973). Botanically, it is the dried flower of the annual herb, 30 to 90 centimeter tall *Carthamus tinctorius* L. of the Compositae family.

Its chemical components are Safflor-yellow and Carthamine (for color). Chinese medicine recognizes its emmenagogal effects and uses it for gynecological disorders such as amenorrhea, dystocia, postpartum hemorrhage, and stagnant blood.

Cassia Seed

CASSIAE TORAE SEMEN
決明子
Chinese Name: (Chyueh-Min-Tzu)

Cassiae Torae Semen is a superior drug recorded in *The Herbal by Shen Nung* (A.D. 25-220). Botanically, it is the dried, ripe seed of the annual herb, the 1 meter tall *Cassia tora* L. of the Leguminosae family.

Its chemical components are emodin, rhein, and chrysophanol. Because of its purgative, refrigerant, and carminative effects, Chinese medicine uses it for headache with fever, eye disorders, ophthalmia with swelling and pain, glaucoma, and dry stools. The cooked seeds can be used as a substitute for tea.

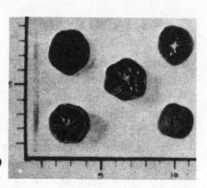

Chih-Shih & Chih-Ko

AURANTII IMMATURUS (BITTER ORANGE)

枳殼　枳實

Chinese Name: (Chih-Ko, Chih-Shih)

Aurantii Immaturus, a general drug recorded in *The Herbal by Shen Nung,* is the dried unripe fruit (Shih) of various oranges (Chih) of the Rutaceae family. The aromatic and bitter fruit is preferred. It is used as an expectorant or as a stomachic for dysentery, tenesmus, and stagnation of food.

The dried and almost ripe fruit of oranges such as *Citrus aurantium* or *C. kotokan* is termed Chih K'o, and the fruit that has been preserved for several years is preferred. It is used for excessive sputum, stomach distention, and abdominal swelling.

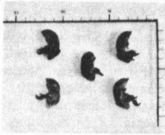

Chrysanthemum

CHRYSANTHEMI FLOS

菊花

Chinese Name: (Chu-Hua)

Chrysanthemi Flos is a superior drug recorded in *The Herbal by Shen Nung* (A.D. 25-220). Botanically, it is the dried flower of the perennial herb, 50 to´ 140 centimeter tall *Chrysanthemum morifloium* Ramat. of the Compositae family.

Because of its purgative and antitoxic effects, Chinese medicine uses it for vertigo, ophthalmia with swelling and pain, and headache with fever. It is also used as a beverage.

Cicade

CICADAE PELLICULA

蟬蛻

Chinese Name: (Chan-Shui)

Cicadae Pellicula, a commonly used drug first recorded in *Ming I Pieh Lu* (A.D. 500), is the dried exuviae of *Cryptotympana atrata* Fabr. of the Cicadidae family.

Chinese medicine recognizes its antipyretic and antispasmodic effects and uses it for headache with fever and convulsions due to fear.

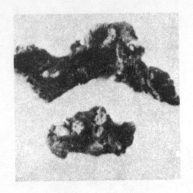

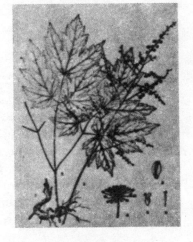

Cimicifuga

CIMICIFUGAE RHIZOMA (MEADOW RUE)

升麻

Chinese Name: (Sheng-Ma)

Cimicifugae Rhizoma, a superior drug recorded in *The Herbal by Shen Nung,* is commonly used in Chinese medicine. Botanically, it is the dried, gray-black, light and durable root-like stem of the perennial two to three-foot tall herb *Cimicifuga heracleifolia, C. dahurica,* or *C. foetida* of the Ranunculaceae family. Since its stem and leaves have the likeness of an ascending (Sheng) hemp (Ma), the plant is named Sheng Ma.

Chinese medicine used Cimicifugae Rhizoma for fever, headache, sore throat, skin eruptions, prolapse of the rectum due to prolonged diarrhea, and metroptosis. Black Snake Root, the North American variation *C. racemosa,* is a folk remedy used for neuralgia and otitis analgesia.

118

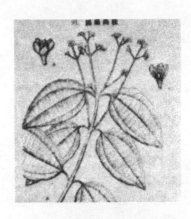

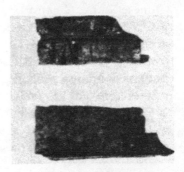

Cinnamon

CINNAMOMI CORTEX AND C. RAMULUS

桂皮　桂枝

Chinese Name: (Kuei-Pi, Kuei-Chih)

Cinnamomi (Kuei) Cortex (Pi), a superior drug recorded in *The Herbal by Shen Nung,* was also recorded as Kassia and Kinnamon in the earliest Western *De Materia Medica* (B.C. 77). In China, it is the dried bark of the twenty to thirty-foot tall *Cinnamomum cassia* Blume and related plants of the Lauraceae family. Cinnamomi (Kuei) Ramulus (Chih) is the dried tender branches of the same plant and has the same applications.

Cinnamomi Cortex and C. Ramulus are generally used as diaphoretics, antipyretics, and analgesics for chills, dizziness, and similar disturbances. Their habitats are China and Vietnam, and their main chemical component is benzaldehyde.

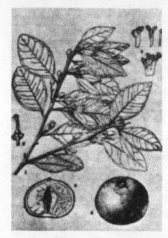

Citrus

CITRUS
RETICULATAE
PERICARPIUM (CITRUS
陳皮   PEEL)
Chinese Name: (Chen-Pi)

Citrus Reticulatae Pericarpium, first recorded as a superior drug in *The Herbal by Shen Nung,* is the peel of the citrus (orange), genus of the Rutaceae family. Because the dried and preserved orange peel is preferred, it possesses the Chinese name Chen (old) Pi (peel).

Chinese medicine uses the peel to arrest vomiting and watery diarrhea, and to relieve chest and abdominal swelling, anorexia, coughs, and excessive phlegm.

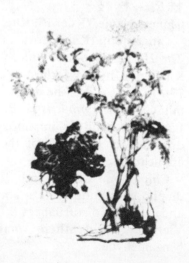

Cnidium

LIGUSTICI
WALLICHII
RHIZOMA (LIGUSTICUM)
川芎
Chinese Name: (Chuan-Chiung)

120

Ligustici Wallichii Rhizoma, a superior drug in *The Herbal by Shen Nung,* is the dried root-like stem of *Ligusticum wallichii* Franch in Taiwan and Hong Kong, and also of *Cnidium officinale* Makino of the Umbelliferae family. In Chinese medicine, it is a gynecological drug used for anemia, scurvy, anxiety, chillphobia, and irregular menstruation.

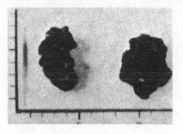

Coix

COICIS SEMEN
(JOB'S TEARS)

薏苡仁

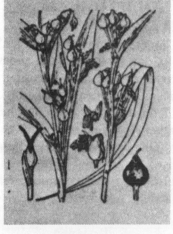

Chinese Name: (I-Yi-Jen)

Coicis Semen, recorded in various Chinese medical texts, is the seeds of an annual, spring-growing, three to four-foot tall herb *Coix lachryma-jobi* L. of the Gramineae family.

In Chinese medicine, Coicis Semen is often used in conjunction with Discoreae Radix, Nelumbinis Semen, Poria, and pig's intestine. These are called the "Four Wonders" 四神 and are used for childhood malnutrition. Coicis Semen alone is used for dysuria, weak stomach, pulmonary tuberculosis, inflammation, pus, pain, and edema. Women use it to relieve dry skin. Its main chemical component is the fatty acid coixenolide.

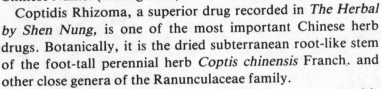

Coptis

COPTIDIS RHIZOMA (GOLDTHREAD)
黃連

Chinese Name: (Huang-Lien)

Coptidis Rhizoma, a superior drug recorded in *The Herbal by Shen Nung,* is one of the most important Chinese herb drugs. Botanically, it is the dried subterranean root-like stem of the foot-tall perennial herb *Coptis chinensis* Franch. and other close genera of the Ranunculaceae family.

This drug is an anti-inflammatory, bitter-tasting stomachic used for internal heat, toxicity, edema, fever and thirst, chest distention and vomiting, febrile dysentery, abdominal ache, anxiety, hemoptysis, nosebleed, and insomnia.

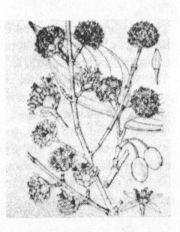

Cornus

CORNI FRUCTUS
山茱萸

Chinese Name: (Shan-Shu-Yu)

Corni Fructus, a general drug recorded in *The Herbal by Shen Nung,* is the fruit (dried and with seeds removed) of the deciduous, 10-foot tall tree, *Cornus officinalis* Sieb. et Zucc. of the Cornaceae family.

Corni Fructus has been used as an astringent, and is a potent drug for menorrhagia, polyuria, continuous perspiration, impotence, nocturnal emission, dizziness, and tinnitus. Cornus or Dogwood Bark, the skin of the root of an American genus *Cornus florida*, L. is often used for weakness, excess moisture, and irregular menstruation.

Corydalis

CORYDALIDIS TUBER

延胡索

Chinese Name: (Yen-Hu-So)

Corydalidis Tuber is a commonly used drug first recorded in *Kai Pao Pen Tsao* (A.D. 973). Botanically, it is the dried tuber of the perennial herb, the 20-centimeter tall *Corydalis ambigua* (Pallas) Chamisso et Schlechtendal, or *Corydalis bulbosa* DC., or other genera of the Papaveraceae family.

Its chemical components are corydaline, dehydro-corydaline, protopine, and coryhulbine. It can be used as a analgesic for headache, abdominal pain, and menstrual cramps. It can stop uterine bleeding, dispel stagnant blood, and improve blood circulation.

Curcuma

CURCUMAE RADIX

鬱金

Chinese Name: (Yu-Chin)

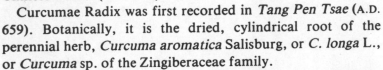

Curcumae Radix was first recorded in *Tang Pen Tsae* (A.D. 659). Botanically, it is the dried, cylindrical root of the perennial herb, *Curcuma aromatica* Salisburg, or *C. longa* L., or *Curcuma* sp. of the Zingiberaceae family.

About six percent of it is composed of the following essential oils: sesquiterpene ($C_{15}H_{24}$), sesquiterpenealcohol, camphor, camphene, and curcumin. It can expel stagnant blood and may be used as a stomachic, analgesic, emmenagogue, and hemostatic agent. Chinese medicine uses it for pain in the chest and abdomen, gallstones, jaundice, hemoptysis, epistaxis, hematuria, epilepsy, menstrual cramps, and fever with sweating.

Cuscuta

CUSCUTAE SEMEN

菟絲子

Chinese Name: (Tu-Szu-Tzu)

Cuscutae Semen is a superior drug recorded in *The Herbal by Shen Nung* (A.D. 25-220). Botanically, it is the dried, ripe seed of the parasitic plant, *Cuscuta chinensis* Lam., or *C. japonica* Choisy of the Convolvulaceae family.

Because of its nutritive, tonic, aphrodisiac, and antidiarrheal effects, Chinese medicine uses it for pain near the waist and in the knees, spermatorrhea, enuresis, and diarrhea.

Cyperus

CYPERI RHIZOMA
香附
Chinese Name: (Shiang-Fu)

Cyperi Rhizoma, originally named Sha-Tsao, is a general drug recorded in *Ming I Pieh Lu* (A.D. 500). Later, it was called Shiang-Fu-Tzu in *Tang Pen Tsao* (A.D. 659). Botanically, it is the dried tuber of the perennial herb, *Cyperus rotundus* L. of the Cyperaceae family.

Because of its emmenagogal, antitussive, antispasmodic, and analgesic effects, Chinese medicine uses it for cough due to tuberculosis, and for uterine disorders, distension and pain in the chest and abdomen, menstrual irregularities, and menstrual cramps.

Dioscorea

DIOSCOREAE RADIX (YAM)
山藥

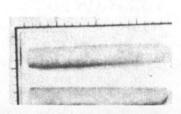

Chinese Name: (Shan-Yao)

Dioscoreae Radix, a superior drug recorded in *The Herbal by Shen Nung,* is also entered in the oldest Western *De*

Materia Medica. Botanically, it is the dried root (with the bark removed) of the perennial, wild or cultivated creeping plant *Dioscorea batatas* Decne or other species of the Dioscoreae family.

Japanese often grind the raw Dioscoreae Radix, then take it with rice. Each gram of the root contains mucin (a mixture of protein and sugar), 0.2 mg. of vitamin B1, 10 to 15 mg. of Vitamin C. It is a tonic and antidysenteric, and is used in Chinese medicine for prolonged diarrhea, weakness and loss of weight, nocturnal emission, leucorrhea, and polyuria.

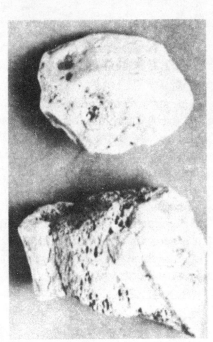

Dragon-Bone

DRACONIS OS
(DRAGON BONE)
龍骨

Chinese Name: (Lung-Ku)

Draconis Os, a superior drug recorded in *The Herbal by Shen Nung,* is the fossilized remains of large mammals such as elephant, deer, or others. It possesses sedative and astringent effects, and is used in Chinese medicine for fright, nightmares, spermatorrhea, epilepsy, leucorrhea with or without blood, prolapse of the rectum, and nosebleed.

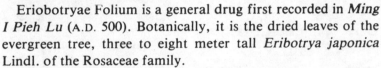

Eriobotrya

ERIOBOTRYAE FOLIUM
枇杷葉

Chinese Name: (Pi-Pa-Yeh)

Eriobotryae Folium is a general drug first recorded in *Ming I Pieh Lu* (A.D. 500). Botanically, it is the dried leaves of the evergreen tree, three to eight meter tall *Eribotrya japonica* Lindl. of the Rosaceae family.

Chinese medicine takes into account its antipyretic, expectorant, antitussive, and diuretic actions and uses it for cough, expectoration with fever, internal heat in the stomach, vomiting, dysuria, and thirst.

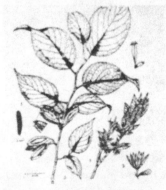

Eucommia

EUCOMMIAE CORTEX
杜仲

Chinese Name: (Tu-Chung)

Eucommiae Cortex is a superior drug recorded in *The Herbal by Shen Nung* (A.D. 25-220). Botanically, it is the dried bark of the deciduous tree, ten-meter tall *Eucommia ulmoides* Oliv. of the Eucommiaceae family.

Because of its nutritive, tonic, analgesic, and sedative effects, Chinese medicine uses it for pain near the waist and in the knees, itching due to moisture in the genital areas, enuresis, and quieting of uterine contractions during pregnancy.

Euryale

EURYALES SEMEN (WATER LILY)
芡實
Chinese Name: (Chien-Shih)

Euryales Semen, a superior drug recorded in *The Herbal by Shen Nung,* is the dried ripe seeds of the water plant *Euryale ferox* Salisb., Nymphaeaceae family. It is a potent drug for treatment of spermatorrhea, leucorrhea, watery diarrhea, inconsistent urination, numbness and aching near the waist and in the knees.

Evodia

EVODIAE FRUCTUS
吳茱萸
Chinese Name: (Wu-Shu-Yu)

Evodiae Fructus is a general drug recorded in *The Herbal by Shen Nung* (A.D. 25-220). Botanically, it is the dried, raw fruit of the woody shrub, the 2.4 to 5-centimeter tall *Evodia rutaecarpa* (Jussieu) Bentham of the Rutaceae family.

Because of its stomachiac, analgesic, and diuretic effects, Chinese medicine uses it to alleviate nausea, vomiting, diarrhea, abdominal distension and pain, menstrual cramps, rheumatic pain, and gastric disorders.

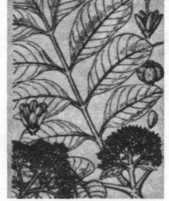

Forsythia

FORSYTHIAE FRUCTUS (GOLDEN BELL)
連翹

Chinese Name: (Lien-Chiao)

Forsythiae Fructus, an inferior drug recorded in *The Herbal by Shen Nung,* is the dried ripe fruit of the cultivated, small, deciduous shrub *Forsythia suspensa* Vahl. and other genera of the Oleaceae family.

Since ancient times, Forsythiae Fructus has been used for its cooling, antiphlogistic, laxative, diuretic, emmenagogue, and pus-discharging functions. Chinese medicine, therefore, uses it for erysipelas, febrile gonorrhea, skin eruptions, scrofula, and carbuncle. It can also be applied externally for scabies.

129

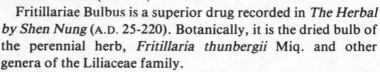

Fritallaria

FRITILLARIAE BULBUS
貝母

Chinese Name: (Pei-Mu)

Fritillariae Bulbus is a superior drug recorded in *The Herbal by Shen Nung* (A.D. 25-220). Botanically, it is the dried bulb of the perennial herb, *Fritillaria thunbergii* Miq. and other genera of the Liliaceae family.

Its chemical components are fritilline, fritillarine, and verticine. It is used as an antitussive, expectorant, and purgative. Chinese medicine gives it for lung disorders in which there is internal heat in the lungs, cough, and expectoration.

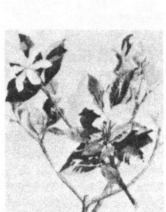

Gardenia

GARDENIAE FRUCTUS (GARDENIA)
栀子

Chinese Name: (Chih-Tzu)

Gardeniae Fructus, a general drug in *The Herbal by Shen Nung,* is the dried ripe fruit of the cultivated, temperate, evergreen, 10-foot shrub *Gardenia jasminosides* Ellis, Rubiaceae family.

Chinese medicine considers it to have anti-inflammatory, antipyretic, astringent, and hemostatic functions. It is used for congestion, nosebleed, hemoptysis, and jaundice. Besides, it is sometimes used for gulletitis, chest and stomach ache, stomatitis, tonsillitis, and mastitis. The main component of its yellow pigment is crocin which is now generally used as a natural yellow pigment.

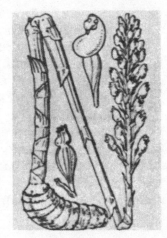

Gastrodia

GASTRODIAE RHIZOMA

天麻

Chinese Name: (Tien-Ma)

Gastrodiae Rhizoma, originally named Chih-Chien, is a superior drug recorded in *The Herbal by Shen Nung* (A.D. 25-220). Later, it was called Tien-Ma in *Kai Pao Pen Tsao* (A.D. 973). Botanically, it is the dried, tuberous root of the parasitic perennial herb with a simple and erect stem, 60 to 100 centimeter tall *Gastrodia elata* Bl. of the Orchidaceae family.

Because of its carminative and antispasmodic effects, Chinese medicine uses it for headache, vertigo, epilepsy, monoplegia, spasms in the arms and legs, and pain in the waist and knees.

131

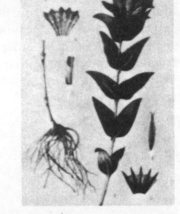

Gentiana

GENTIANAE RADIX

龍膽

Chinese Name: (Lung-Tan)

Gentianae Radix is a general drug recorded in *The Herbal by Shen Nung* (A.D. 25-220). Botanically, it is the dried root of the perennial herb, the 30 to 60 centimeter tall *Gentiana scabra* Bunge, and other genera of the Gentianaceae family.

The roots are officinal, and they have a bitter taste. Their primary chemical component is gentiopicyin which dissolves in water to produce gentiogenin and glucose. This drug is a bitter stomachic, carminative, and purgative agent. Chinese medicine uses it for chills, fever, agitated epilepsy, intercostal neuralgia, ophthalmia, sore throat, bitter taste in the mouth, and swelling carbuncles.

Ginger

ZINGIBERIS (RECENS) RHIZOMA (GINGER)

生薑　乾薑

Chinese Name: (Sheng-Chiang, Kan-Chiang)

132

Zingiberis Recens Rhizoma, 生薑 a general drug recorded in *The Herbal by Shen Nung,* is the fresh, root-like stem of the perennial, two to three-foot tall *Zingiber officinale* Rosc. of the Zingiberaceae family cultivated in tropical and temperate regions. (Z. Rhizoma is the sun-dried.) Its acrid components arc known as zingerone, shogaol, and gingerone and are used in stomachics.

Because of the different times of collection and varying processes, the effects of the two herbs differ somewhat. Zingiberis Recens Rhizoma (Sheng-Chiang) is an aromatic stomachic mainly used for a cold due to wind-chill, for nausea and vomiting, and for stridor. Z. Rhizoma (Kan-Chiang) is used mainly for vomiting and diarrhea, abdominal ache, rheumatism, and ache in the spleen or abdomen.

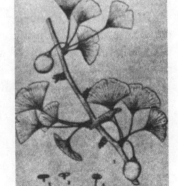

Ginkgo

GINKGO SEMEN
白果　　　　銀杏
Chinese Name: (Pai-Kuo)

Ginkgo Semen, originally named Yin-Hsing, is a commonly used drug recorded in *Tze Yeou Pen Tsao* (A.D. 1328-1329). Botanically, it is the dried, ripe seed (exclusive of the fleshy epidermis) of the deciduous tree, the 40 meter tall *Ginkgo biloba* L. of the Ginkoaceae family.

It may be used as a food. Chinese medicine recognizes its astringent, sedative, and antitussive effects and uses it for persistent cough, wheezing, spermatorrhea, and frequent micturition.

133

Ginseng

GINSENG RADIX
(GINSENG)

人参

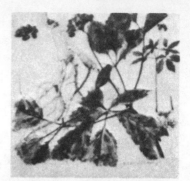

Chinese Name: (Jen-Sheng)

Ginseng Radix, a superior drug of *The Herbal by Shen Nung,* has been a tonic highly valued by Chinese and Japanese. Botanically, it is the dried root of the perennial, foot-tall herb *Panax ginseng* C. A. Meyer of the Araliaceae family which grows mainly in Korea and Japan. Because it has the shape of a man, the root is called Jen (man's) Sheng (tonic).

Ginseng Radix, a nutritive tonic, is used mainly for improving a delicate physique, weakness during convalescence, neurasthenia, impotence, spermatorrhea, senility, anemia, nephritis, and uterine diseases.

Gypsum

FIBROSUM
GYPSUM

石膏

Chinese Name: (Shih-Kao)

Fibrosum Gypsum, a general medicine recorded in *The Herbal by Shen Nung,* is the mineral, hydrated calcium sulfate, $CaSO_4$-$2H_2O$, occurring naturally in sedimentary rocks in bays or rivers. Because of its cooling and thirst quenching effects, Chinese medicine uses it for thirst, fever, dizziness, stridor, and sunstroke.

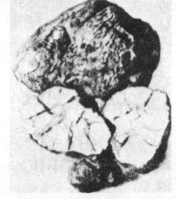

Hoelen

PORIA (INDIAN BREAD)
茯苓
Chinese Name: (Fu-Ling)

Poria, one of the most important diuretics, is recorded in various herbal texts. Botanically, it is generally the *Poria cocos* Wolf., with a dark-brown outer layer and a white inner part, which is parasitic on pine and weighs up to 2 kg. in a fruiting body. Chinese medicine uses it to balance body fluids increase urinary volume, to dispel stagnant water in the stomach, and to treat tachycardia.

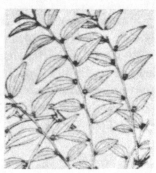

Jujube

ZIZYPHI SEMEN
酸棗仁
Chinese Name: (Shuan-Tsao-Jen)

Zizyphi Semen is a superior drug recorded in *The Herbal by Shen Nung* (A.D. 25-220). Botanically, it is the dried, ripe seed of the deciduous tree, one to three meter tall *Zizyphus jujuba* Mill. var *spinosa* Hu of the Rhamnaceae family.

Its chemical components are Betulin and Betulinic acid, and it is used as a nutritive tonic, sedative, and stomachic. Chinese medicine gives it for insomnia due to stress, palpitations due to anxiety, amnesia, thirst, weakness, and ephidrosis.

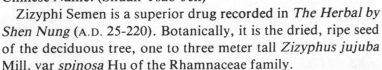

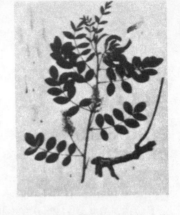

Licorice

GLYCYRRHIZAE RADIX (LICORICE)

甘草

Chinese Name: (Kan-Tsao)

Glycyrrhizae Radix, a very commonly used Chinese herb is also recorded in the works of the Greek Theophrastus (B.C. 372-287), as well as in the pharmacopoeias of various countries. Botanically, it is the root of the perennial herb *Glycyrrhiza uralensis* Fisch. et DC. and other genera *G. glabra*, L. *G. echinata*, and *G. glabra* var. *glandulifera* of the Leguminosae family grown in China (Northwest provinces and Mongolia) and Pakistan. The root tastes very sweet; therefore, it is called Kan (sweet) Tsao (herb).

Western countries use Glycyrrhizae Radix mainly as a corrigent. Chinese medicine uses it for toxic states, excessive sputum, muscular pain due to tension, peptic ulcer, duodenal ulcer, and sore throat. The sweet components are mainly glycyrrhizin.

Lindera

LINDERAE RADIX

烏藥

Chinese Name: (Wu-Yao)

136

Linderae Radix is a commonly used drug recorded in *Kai Pao Pen Tsao* (A.D. 973) of the Sung Dynasty. Botanically, it is the dried root of the aromatic shrub, the four to five meter tall *Lindera strychnifolia* F. Vill. of the Lauraceae family.

Its chemical components are linderane, linderene, and linderene acetate, and it is an aromatic with stomachic, and analgesic effects. Chinese medicine uses it for pain and distension in the chest, nausea and vomiting, frequent micturition, and hernia.

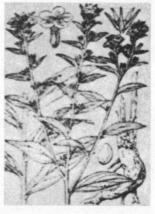

Lithospermum

LITHOSPERMI RADIX
紫根
Chinese Name: (Tzu-Ken)

Lithospermi Radix, a superior drug recorded in *The Herbal by Shen Nung*, is the root (Ken) of a purplish (Tsu) herb. Botanically, it is the root of the perennial, two to three-foot tall *Lithosperum officinale L.* or *L. officinale* var. *erythrorhizon* Maxim of the Boraginaceae family.

Chinese medicine considers its antipyretic, detoxifying, and purgative effects, and uses it for skin eruptions, swelling, and dry stool and constipation. It is the principal constituent of Lithospermium Ointment, widely recognized as the best external Chinese drug to regenerate skin tissue. For the past 350 years the ointment has been generally and effectively used for skin eruptions, burns, chilblain, and hemorrhoids.

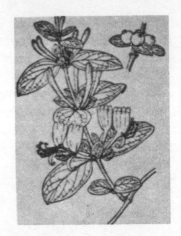

Lonicera

LONICERAE FLOS

金銀花

Chinese Name: (Chin-Yin-Hua)

Lonicerae Flos is a commonly used drug first recorded in *Pen Tsao Kang Mu* (A.D. 1593). Botanically, it is the dried flower of the perennial, volubilate shrub, the 9-meter tall *Lonicera japonica* Thunb. of the Caprifoliaceae family.

Because of its antipyretic, antitoxic, and refrigerant effects, Chinese medicine uses it for fever of the warm diseases, and for swelling carbuncles and scabies.

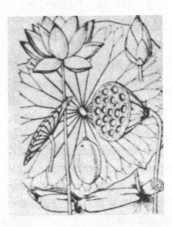

Lotus Seed

NELUMBINIS SEMEN (EAST INDIAN LOTUS)

蓮子

Chinese Name: (Lien-Tzu)

Nelumbinis Semen, a drug recorded in *The Herbal by Shen Nung,* is the dried ripe seeds of the pond and swamp waterplant, *Nelumbo nucifera* Gaertn., Nymphaeaceae family. Being a tonic for the heart and viscera, it is used for weak spleen, watery diarrhea, nightmares, spermatorrhea, metrorrhagia, and leucorrhea. In Chinese medicine, the embryos are removed before the seeds are used.

Lotus Stamen

LOTI STAMEN
蓮鬚

Chinese Name: (Lien-Hsu)

Loti Stamen is recorded in *Pen Tsao Kang Mu* (A.D. 1593). Botanically, it is the dried stamen of the perennial, aquatic plant, *Nelumbo nucifera* Gaertn. of the Nymphaeaceae family.

Because of its astringent, hemostatic, nutritive, and tonic effects, Chinese medicine uses it for spermatorrhea and hemoptysis.

Lycium Fruit

LYCII FRUCTUS
枸杞子

Chinese Name: (Kou-Chi-Tzu)

Lycii Fructus is a superior drug recorded in *The Herbal by Shen Nung* (A.D. 25-220). Botanically, it is the dried, ripe fruit of the 1-meter tall shrub. *Lycium barbarum* L., or *Lycium Chinese Mill.*, of the Solanaceae family.

Chinese medicine recognizes its nutritive and tonic effects and uses it for weaknesses of the liver and kidneys, aching near the waist and in the knees, and vertigo.

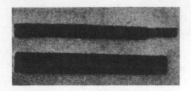

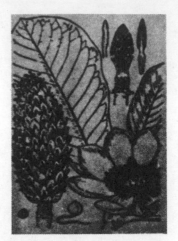

Magnolia Bark

MAGNOLIAE CORTEX
厚朴

Chinese Name: (Hou-Pu)

Magnoliae Cortex is the dried trunk or root-bark of the wild, deciduous, forty to fifty-foot tall mountain tree *Magnolia officinalis* Rehd. et Wils. or *M. officinalis* var. *biloba* Rehd. et Wils. of the Magnoliaceae family in China. The bark is thick (Hou), and its composition plain and simple (Pu). In Japan, however, *M. obovata* Thunb of the same genus is used.

Chinese medicine uses it as a stomachic and astringent for dysuria, visceral distension, abdominal pain, and cough. Magnocurarine and Magnonol, its main components, are bacteriostatic and bacteriocidal.

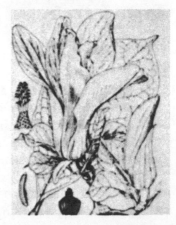

Magnolia Flower

MAGNOLIAE LILIFLORAE FLOS (MAGNOLIA)
辛夷

Chinese Name: (Hsin-I)

Magnoliae Liliflorae Flos, also called Spring Flower, is a general drug of *The Herbal by Shen Nung*. Botanically, it is the buds of the deciduous tree *Magnolia liliflora* Desr. and its close species of the same genus of the Magnoliaceae family. In China and Japan, it is used as a sedative and analgesic for headache, rhinitis, and suppuration. Clinical experiments have used the Magnoliae Liliflorae Flos preparations in the treatment of nasal catarrh.

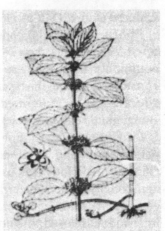

Mentha

MENTHAE HERBA (PEPPERMINT)
薄荷

Chinese Name: (Po-Ho)

Menthae Herba, a most commonly used drug first recorded in *Sin Siu Pen Tsao* (New Revision of The Herbal) in A.D. 659, was used by Western medicine in Europe during the 18th century. Botanically, it is the dried stem and leaves of the perennial, two-foot herb *Mentha arvensis* var. *piperascens* Holmes of the Labiatae family grown in the Orient.

Chinese physicians consider Menthae Herba's digestive and heat-dispersing effects, and often use it for colds, fever, headache, laryngeal swelling and weak stomach. Distillation of the herb will produce peppermint oil, an essential oil used in the making of menthol biscuits and dental plates (dentures).

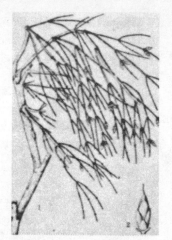

M. H. (Ephedra)

EPHEDRA HERBA
(EPHEDRA)
麻黄

Chinese Name: (Ma-Huang)

Ephedrae Herba, a general drug recorded in *The Herbal by Shen Nung,* has been one of the best-known and most commonly used Chinese herb drugs. Botanically, it is now considered to be the spring growth of the shrubs *Ephedra sinica* Stapf, *E. intermedia* Schrenk et Meyer, *E. equisetina* Bunge, and related species of the Ephedraceae family.

In ancient times, Ephedra Herba was used to increase perspiration and to treat fever, cough, and dysuria. Now Chinese medicine often uses it for bronchial asthma, urticaria, and cough, while Western medicine uses it only for bronchial asthma. Its main chemical component is ephedrine. Only the internodes are used; the nodes of the stem are discarded.

Mirabilitum

DEPURATUM
MIRABILITUM
芒硝

Chinese Name: (Mang Hsiao)

Depuratum Mirabilitum, a superior drug recorded in *The Herbal by Shen Nung,* is the processed crystals of natural sodium sulfate, Na2SO4. However, Japanese scholars have analyzed the Depuratum Mirabilitum that has been preserved since the Tang Dynasty of China at the Shosoin Treasure House in Nara, Japan, and they discovered that these crystals are magnesium sulfate, MgSO4.

Chinese medicine has considered this drug to be effective in moistening, urination, softening, and purgation, and has used it for gastrointestinal fever and stagnation, dry stools and constipation, and jaundice.

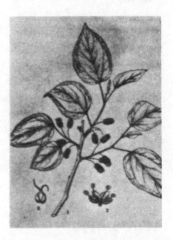

Morus

MORI CORTEX
桑白皮

Chinese Name: (Sang-Pai-Pi)

Mori Cortex is a general drug first recorded in *The Herbal by Shen Nung* (A.D. 25-220). Botanically, it is the epidermis of the dried root, *Morus alba* Linne of the Moraceae family.

Its chemical components are b-Amyrin, Sitosterol, and Resinotannol. It is given as a diuretic, antiphlogistic, and antitussive. Chinese medicine uses it for asthma, cough, internal heat in the lungs, hemoptysis, anascara, and abdominal distension.

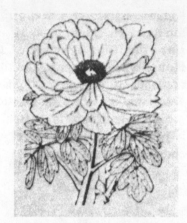

Moutan

MOUTAN RADICIS CORTEX (TREE PEONY)
牡丹皮

Chinese Name: (Mu-Tan-Pi)

Moutan Radicis Cortex, a superior drug recorded in *The Herbal by Shen Nung,* is the dried root-bark of the deciduous, two to three-foot tall *Paeonia suffruticosa* Andr. of the Ranunculaceae family. The plant has very beautiful flowers and a particular fragrance that makes it a desirable garden flower in China.

Chinese medicine uses the drug mainly for inflammation, pain-relief, stagnant blood, and gynecopathy. Its main chemical component, paeonol, has antibacterial action.

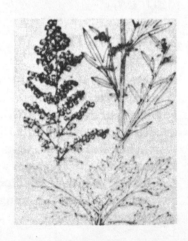

Mugwort
(Artemisia leaves)

ARTEMISIAE ARGYI FOLIUM (WORMWOOD)
艾葉

Chinese Name: (Ai-Yeh)

Artemisiae Argyi Folium, also known as the herb of moxibustion, or the leaf of moxa, is recorded in *Ming I Pieh Lu* (Reference of Reputed Physicians). Botanically, it is the dried leaf of *Artemisia argyi* Levl. et Vant. of the Compositae family in China, but of *A. vulgaris* L. var. *indica* maxim or *A. montana* in Japan.

Considering its hemostatic, astringent, menstrual, and fetus-stabilizing effects, Chinese medicine uses Artemisiae Argyi Folim for irregular menstruation, leucorrhea with or without blood, unstable fetus, prolonged diarrhea, hemoptysis, nosebleed, and as an assistant drug for gynecopathy. Its principal chemical constituents are adenine, cineol, and various vitamins.

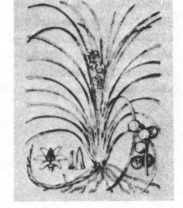

Ophiopogon

OPHIOPOGONIS RADIX

麥門冬

Chinese Name: (Mai-Men-Tung)

Ophiopogonis Radix is a superior drug recorded in *The Herbal by Shen Nung* (A.D. 25-220). Botanically, it is the dried root of the perennial herb, the fifteen to forty centimeter tall *Ophiopogon japonicus* Ker-Gawl. of the Liliaceae family.

Its chemical components are b-sitosterol, stigmasterol, and vitamin A. Chinese medicine recognizes its salivant, nutritive, expectorant, antitussive, and diuretic effects and uses it for cough, hemoptysis, thirst, dysuria, and weakness due to stress.

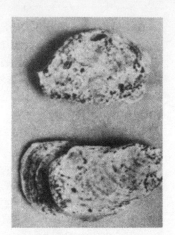

Ostrea tests

OSTREAE CONCHA
牡蠣

Chinese Name: (Mu-Li)

Ostreae Concha, a superior drug recorded in *The Herbal by Shen Nung,* is the soft-bodied invertebrate and shell of *Ostrea rivularis* and a wide source of all others in the Ostreidae family. Chinese medicine takes into account its astringent and sedative effects, and uses it for fatigue, anxiety, sweating, night sweats, nocturnal emission, leucorrhea, and gastro-intestinal hyperacidity. Its main chemical components are calcium carbonate and calcium phosphate.

Paeonia

PAEONIAE ALBA
RADIX (PEONY)
白芍

Chinese Name: (Pai-Shao)

Paeoniae Alba Radix, mentioned in various Chinese herbal texts, is also a garden flower like Moutan Radicis Cortex (Tree Peony). Botanically, it is the dried, cork-removed root of the perennial one to two-foot *Paeonia lactiflora* Pall. of the Ranunculaceae family.

146

Because of its antispasmodic and analgesic effects, Chinese medicine uses it for gastrospasm, abdominal ache, neuralgia, and painful and irregular menstruation. Its known chemical components, paeoniflorin and two similar compounds, have shown sedative and analgesic properties in clinical experiments. Paeoniac Rubra Radix retains the cork and has similar effects.

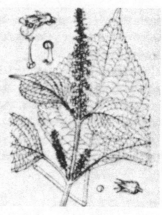

Perilla

PERILLAE ACUTAE FOLIUM
紫蘇葉

Chinese Name: (Tzu-Su-Yeh)

Perillae Acutae Folium is the dried leaves of the annual, two to three-foot tall *Perilla frutescens* var. *crispa* Decne. of the Labiatae family. The leaves (Yeh) are red-purple (Tzu) and have a dilating (Su) property, and is thus called Tzu-Su-Yeh.

Chinese medicine uses the leaves to stimulate perspiration and as treatment for fever, common cold, cough, wheezing, and abdominal distention. It may also be used as a flavoring agent in the manufacture of foods and biscuits. Its main chemical component is perilla-aldehyde.

147

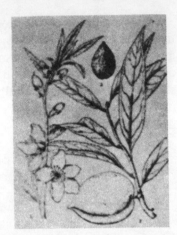

Persica

PERSICAE SEMEN (PEACH SEED)

桃仁

Chinese Name: (Tao-Jen)

Persicae Semen, or peach (Tao) kernel (Jen) as recorded in *The Herbal by Shen Nung,* is the seed of our fruit. Botanically, it is the seeds of the perennial, deciduous, over ten-foot tall tree, *Prunus persica* Batsch or *P. davidiana* Carr., Rosaceae family.

Chinese medicine uses Persicae Semen as an antiphlogistic and antistagnant blood agent to relieve lower abdominal ache, irregular menstruation, intestinal obstruction, carbuncles, dry stools, and constipation. Like Armeniacae Amarae Semen (Apricot Seed), its main chemical component is amygdalin and the fragrance of benzaldehyde.

Peucedanum

PEUCEDANI RADIX

前胡

Chinese Name: (Chien-Hu)

Peucedani Radix is a general drug recorded in *Ming I Pieh Lu* (A.D. 500). Botanically, it is the dried root of the perennial

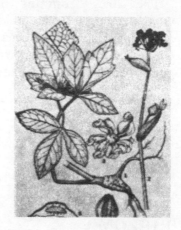

herb, *Peucedanum Praeruptorum* Dunn., or *P. decursivum* Maxim. of the Umbelliferae family.

It contains the glycoside nodakenin and is an analgesic, antitussive, and expectorant. Chinese medicine uses it for the common cold, cough, chest distension, viscid sputum, asthma, vomiting, and nausea.

Phellodendron

PHELLODENDRI CORTEX
黃蘗

Chinese Name: (Huang-Po)

Phellodendri Cortex, originally named Po-Mu, is a general drug first recorded in *The Herbal by Shen Nung* (A.D. 25-220). It is called Huang-Po in *Ming I Pieh Lu* (A.D. 400). Botanically, it is the dried bark of the deciduous tree, the ten to fifteen meter tall *Phellodendron amurense* Rupr., or *P. chinense* Schneid. of the Rutaceae family.

The drug contains Berberine, Phelloderine, and Obakulactone. It is used as a bitter stomachic and antiphlogistic, mainly because of the action of berberine. Chinese medicine gives it for diarrhea with fever, jaundice, gonorrhea, hemorrhoids, and melena.

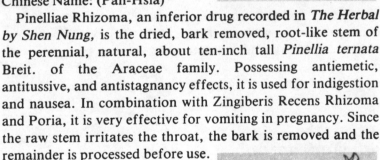

Pinellia

PINELLIAE RHIZOMA (PINELLIA)
半夏
Chinese Name: (Pan-Hsia)

Pinelliae Rhizoma, an inferior drug recorded in *The Herbal by Shen Nung,* is the dried, bark removed, root-like stem of the perennial, natural, about ten-inch tall *Pinellia ternata* Breit. of the Araceae family. Possessing antiemetic, antitussive, and antistagnancy effects, it is used for indigestion and nausea. In combination with Zingiberis Recens Rhizoma and Poria, it is very effective for vomiting in pregnancy. Since the raw stem irritates the throat, the bark is removed and the remainder is processed before use.

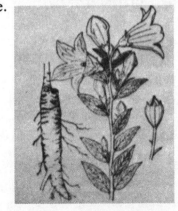

Platycodon

PLATYCODI RADIX (KIKIA ROOT)
桔梗
Chinese Name: (Chie-Keng)

Platycodi Radix, an inferior drug recorded in *The Herbal by Shen Nung,* is the dried root of the perennial, over one-foot tall herb, *Platycodon grandiflorum A. DC. (P. glaucum)* of the Campanulaceae family. The plant grows in the frigid and temperate zones of Asia—mainly Korea—and blossoms in beautiful purple and white bell flowers in the spring.

Chinese medicine uses Platycodi Radix for sore throat, cough, tonsilitis, suppuration, and suppurative bronchitis. Its main chemical component, Kikyo-saponin which increases tracheal secretions, has an expectorant effect.

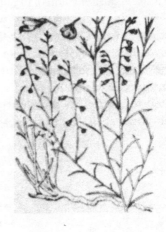

Polygala

POLYGALAE RADIX (CHINESE LENEGA)

遠志

Chinese Name: (Yuan-Chih)

Polygalae Radix, also called "Small Herb," is a superior drug of *The Herbal by Shen Nung.* Botanically, it is the root of the perennial, nine to ten-inch tall, slender leaf herb, *Polygala tenuifolia* Willd., or *P. senega* L. of the North America and Canada, of the Polygalaceae family.

Both genera contain a saponin that helps discharge sputum. Western medicine uses Polygalae Radix in the manufacture of expectorants. Chinese medicine, in addition to using it as an expectorant, considers it a brain tonic and uses it for fright, amnesia, nightmares, and insomnia.

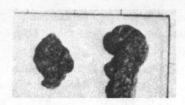

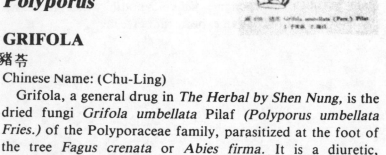

Polyporus

GRIFOLA

豬苓

Chinese Name: (Chu-Ling)

Grifola, a general drug in *The Herbal by Shen Nung,* is the dried fungi *Grifola umbellata* Pilaf *(Polyporus umbellata Fries.)* of the Polyporaceae family, parasitized at the foot of the tree *Fagus crenata* or *Abies firma.* It is a diuretic, antipyretic, and thirst-quencher in Chinese medicine, and is used for difficulty in urination, for edema and distension, and for gonorrhea, leucorrhea, and hematuria.

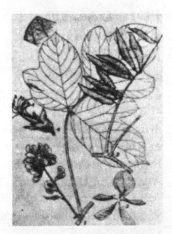

Pueraria

PUERARIAE
RADIX
(PUERARIA)

葛根

Chinese Name: (Ko-Ken)

Puerariae Radix, a general drug of *The Herbal by Shen Nung,* is the main herb used in the Pueraria Combination.

Botanically, it is the root of the perennial, wild, creeping herb, *Pueraria pseudo-hirsuta* Tang et Wang or another species of the Leguminosae family.

The root contains a large percentage of the starch puerariae amylum, which may be used as a binder and an ingredient in the making of biscuits. In addition, its main component, daidzein, has antispasmodic and antipyretic effects. It is used for fever, thirst, diarrhea, and skin eruptions.

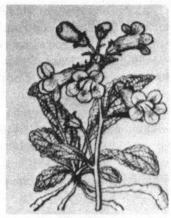

Rehmannia

REHMANNIAE RADIX (REHMANNIA)

地黃

Chinese Name: (Ti-Huang)

Rehmanniae Radix, a very commonly used drug recorded in *The Herbal by Shen Nung* and of the same family as Digitalis, is the root-like stem of the perennial, seven to eight-inch tall herb, *Rehmannia glutinosa* Libosch of the Scrophulariaceae family. The sun-dried root-like stem is called "Dried Rehmanniae Radix" and the one stored in sand "Raw Rehmanniae Radix." Chinese medicine uses it as a hematinic for anemia, hemoptysis, impotence, weakness, and spermatorrhea. It often appears in the formulas for gynecopathy.

153

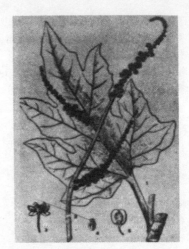

Rhubarb

RHEI RHIZOMA (RHUBARB)
大黃
Chinese Name: (Ta-Huang)

Rhei Rhizoma, an inferior (toxic) drug recorded in *The Herbal by Shen Nung* and in pharmacopoeias of various countries, is the root-like stem of the perennial, four to five-foot tall herb, *Rheum palmatum* L. and close species of the Polygonaceae family. The plant has large (Ta) leaves and a yellow color (Huang), and it is thus called Ta-Huang. Striped Rhei Rhizoma is preferred.

The herb contains anthraquinone, senoside, emodin, chrysophanic acid, and rhein. It is used as a stomachic and purgative for internal heat, constipation, abdominal ache, mania, edema, amenorrhea, and jaundice.

Saussurea

SAUSSUREAE RADIX
木香
Chinese Name: (Mu-Shiang)

Saussureae Radix is a superior drug recorded in *The Herbal by Shen Nung* (A.D. 25-220). Botanically, it is the dried root of

154

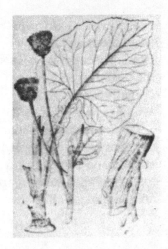

the tall, perennial herb, *Saussurea lappa* Clarke of the Compositae family.

It is used as an aromatic stomachic, vermifuge, and fragrance. Chinese medicine gives it for distension and pain in the chest and abdomen, indigestion, vomiting, diarrhea, tenesmus, and quieting of premature uterine contractions during pregnancy.

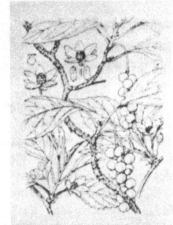

Schizandra

SCHIZANDRAE FRUCTUS (SCHIZANDRA SEEDS)
五味子

Chinese Name: (Wu-Wei-Tzu)

Schizandrae Fructus, a superior drug recorded in *The Herbal by Shen Nung,* is the dried ripe fruit of the evergreen

155

creeping rattan, *Schizandra chinensis* Baillon of the Magnoliaceae family which grows in Japan, Korea, and North China. Because it possesses the five flavors, sweet and sour in the peel and pulp of the fruit, and acrid-bitter and salty in the kernel and salty for the whole. As a result the fruit is thus called Wu (five) Wei (tastes) Tzu (fruit).

Chinese medicine considers its astringent, antitussive, and expectorant effects and uses it for pulmonary weakness, stridor and cough, thirst, night sweats, prolonged diarrhea, insomnia and amnesia, and spermatorrhea. Its main chemical component is Schizandrin.

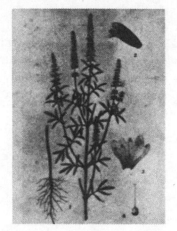

Schizonepeta

SCHIZONEPETAE HERBA (SCHIZONEPETA)

荆芥

Chinese Name: (Chin-Chieh)

Schizonepetae Herba, a general drug recorded in *The Herbal by Shen Nung* and also called Pseudo-Perilla, belongs to the same family as Perillae Herba and Menthae Herba. Botanically, it is the dried herb with flowers of the annual, wild or cultivated, over one-foot tall *Schizonepeta tenuifolia* Brig. of the Labiatae family.

Chinese medicine uses it for the common cold, lack of perspiration, toxic states, headache, fever, sore throat, and scabies. The herb has a special fragrance and contains an essential oil (1% to 2%), which is mainly menthone.

Scute

SCUTELLARIAE RADIX (SKULLCAP)
黃芩

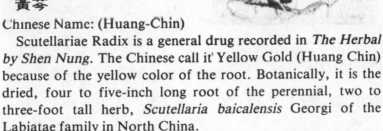

Chinese Name: (Huang-Chin)

Scutellariae Radix is a general drug recorded in *The Herbal by Shen Nung.* The Chinese call it Yellow Gold (Huang Chin) because of the yellow color of the root. Botanically, it is the dried, four to five-inch long root of the perennial, two to three-foot tall herb, *Scutellaria baicalensis* Georgi of the Labiatae family in North China.

Chinese medicine often uses it for various febrile diseases accompanied by such symptoms as red eyes, insomnia, hypertension and headache. It is also used for bleeding, especially nosebleed and hemoptysis. The main chemical components of the root are flavones of baicalin and wagonin.

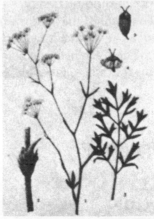

Siler

SILERIS RADIX (SILER)
防風

Chinese Name: (Fang-Feng)

Sileris Radix, a general drug recorded in *The Herbal by Shen Nung,* is the brush-like root of the perennial herb,

Lebebouriella seseloides Wolff and closely related herbs of the Umbelliferae family in N. China. Being a carminative and moderate diaphoretic, it bears the name Fang (prevention against) Feng (wind). Chinese medicine uses it for wind-chill, headache and dizziness, generalized ache, muscle spasm in the limbs, and joint ache.

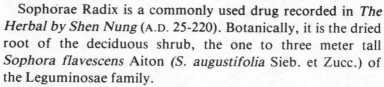

Sophora

SOPHORAE RADIX
苦參

Chinese Name: (Ku-Tsan)

Sophorae Radix is a commonly used drug recorded in *The Herbal by Shen Nung* (A.D. 25-220). Botanically, it is the dried root of the deciduous shrub, the one to three meter tall *Sophora flavescens* Aiton *(S. augustifolia* Sieb. et Zucc.) of the Leguminosae family.

The taste of the root is very bitter. It contains matrine and is used as a stomachic, purgative, diuretic, carminative, and vermifuge. Chinese medicine gives it for diarrhea with bloody stools, jaundice, tabes mesentericus, dysuria, and scabies.

Stephania

STEPHANIAE RADIX
防己

Chinese Name: (Fang-Chi)

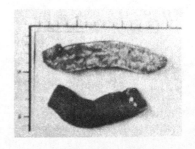

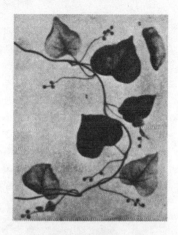

Stephaniae Radix is a general drug recorded in *The Herbal by Shen Nung* (A.D. 25-220). Botanically, it is the dried root of *Stephania tetrandra* S. Moore of the Menispermaceae family.

Its chemical components are tetrandrine, dimethyl tetrandrine, and fanchimoline. It is used as a carminative, diuretic, and purgative. Chinese medicine uses it for edema, inflammation, beriberi, rheumatism, neuralgia, carbuncles, and severe scabies.

Tang-Kuei

ANGELICAE SINENSIS RADIX (ANGELICA, TANG-KUEI)
當歸

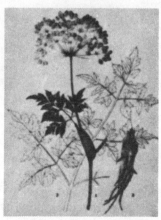

Chinese Name: (Tang-Kuei)

Angelicae Sinensis Radix, a most commonly used Chinese herb drug and a general drug recorded in *The Herbal by Shen Nung,* is a perennial herb with a height of two to three feet in its native mountain habitat. Botanically, it is the dried root of

159

Angelica sinensis (Oliv) Diels or *A. acutiloba* (S. et Z.) Kitag. of the Umbelliferae family.

As an extravasated blood agent, hematinic, sedative, and tonic, Angelicae Sinensis Radix has been used in Chinese medicine for anemia, headache, lumbago, angina and abdominal ache, generalized chills, and menstrual aberrations. Its characteristic fragrance, identified as n-butylidenphthalide, has the sedative component ligustilide.

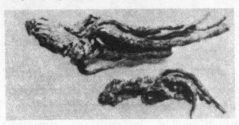

Terminallia

TERMINALIAE FRUCTUS
訶子

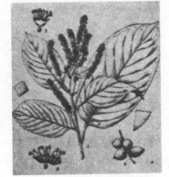

Chinese Name: (Ho-Tzu)

Terminaliae Fructus is a seldom used drug first recorded in *Tang Pen Tsao* (A.D. 659). Botanically, it is the dried, ripe fruit of the deciduous tree, the fifteen to twenty meter tall *Terminalia chebula* Retz. of the Combretaceae family.

The fruit contains tannin (20-40%) and is used as an astringent, expectorant, and antitussive. Chinese medicine gives it for prolonged diarrhea, spermatorrhea, night sweats, and leucorrhea.

Trichosanthes Seed

TRICHOSANTHIS FRUCTUS ET SEMEN

栝樓　栝樓仁

Chinese Name: (Kua-Lou, Kua-Lou-Jen)

Trichosanthis Fructus et Semen is a general herb recorded in *The Herbal by Shen Nung* (A.D. 25-220). Botanically, it is the dried fruit, epidermis, or seed of the perennial vine, *Trichosanthes kirilowii* Maxim. or *T. multiloba* Miq. of the Curcurbitacease family.

The fruit is prescribed as an antitussive, sedative, antipyretic, and diuretic. The kernel is prescribed as an expectorant and as a remedy for dry stools. The epidermis is prescribed as an antipyretic and antitussive and is used to treat thirst, pain due to swelling in the throat, jaundice, anascara, and internal heat in the lungs.

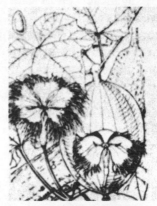

Trichosanthes Root

TRICHOSANTHIS RADIX

栝樓根

Chinese Name: (Kua-Lou-Ken)

Trichosanthis Radix is a general drug first recorded in *Tu Chin Pen Tsao* (A.D. 1062). Botanically, it is the dried root of the perennial vine, *Trichosanthes kirilowii* Maxim. of the Cucurbitaceae family.

The root is considered to have antipyretic, salivant, and antitoxic properties. Chinese medicine uses it for jaundice, febrile diseases, thirst, diabetes, and swollen hemorrhoids.

Tu-huo

ANGELICAE
TUHUO RADIX
獨活

Chinese Name: (Tu-Huo)

Angelicae Tuhuo Radix is the root of a biennial herb which reaches a height of six to seven feet in summer. Because it can stand erect despite the wind, it possesses the name Tuo (alone) Huo (live) in Chinese. Botanically, it is the dried root of *Angelica laxiflora* Diels and its variations of the Umbelliferae family.

Angelicae Tuhuo Radix has chill and moisture dispersing as well as antipruritic functions. It is used in Chinese medicine for head colds, rheumatism, waist and knee aching, and spasm in the limbs. Its principal chemical constituents are angelical and glabra lactone.

Tussilago

FARFARAE FLOS
款冬花

Chinese Name: (Kuan-Tong-Hua)

Farfarae Flos is a general drug recorded in *The Herbal by Shen Nung* (A.D. 25-220). Botanically, it is the dried, young, floral buds of the perennial herb, the ten to twenty-five centimeter tall *Tussilago farfara* L. of Compositae family.

It has antitussive and expectorant effects. Chinese medicine uses it for cough, wheezing, dysphagia, lung disorders, and hemoptysis with pus.

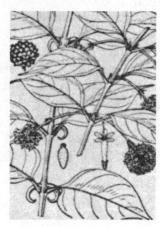

Uncaria (Gambir)

UNCARIAE CUM
UNCIS RAMULUS
鈎藤

Chinese Name: (Kou-Teng)

Uncariae Cum Uncis Ramulus is an inferior drug first recorded in *Ming I Pieh Lu* (A.D. 500). Botanically, it is the dried stem and spines of the evergreen shrub, the one to three meter tall *Uncaria rhynchophylla* (Miq.) Jacks. of the Rubiaceae family.

Because of its antipyretic, antispasmodic, and sedative effects, it is used for infantile febrile diseases, vertigo, hypertension with headache, and epilepsy in children.

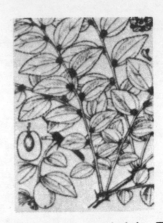

Zizyphus

ZIZPHI SATIVAE FRUCTUS (ZIZYPHUS)
大棗

Chinese Name: (Ta-Tsao)

Zizphi Sativae Fructus, a superior drug recorded in *The Herbal by Shen Nung* and also called the Chinese Date, denotes the big (Ta) and fat dates (sao). The raw fruit may be used as food, while the big and fat fruit collected in autumn and then sun-dried and steam-dried are for medicinal use. Botanically, it belongs to the deciduous, over twenty-foot tall *Zizyphus sativa* or *Z. jujuba* of the Rhamnaceae family in China and to *Z. vulgaris* var. *inermis* in Japan. This fruit contains saccharides, mucus, and malic acid. It is mainly used for weak spleen and stomach, diarrhea, dysentery, and insufficient body fluid. It may also be used for joint spasm, sensitivity, and abdominal ache.

PART IV

Diagnostic Outlines For
The 13 Most Commonly Used
Chinese Formulas

CHINESE
HERB DIAGNOSIS

Chinese medicine, which emphasizes treatment, gives special attention to the patient's pains, or "the conformation." The cardinal principle is that a remedy should be prescribed in accordance with the symptoms, thus a good result can only be expected if the symptoms are properly identified and the medication appropriate to them taken. The following diagrams are for the thirteen most commonly used Chinese prescriptions. On these diagrams the *principal* symptoms are indicated by sans serif type set in all capital letters, and the *secondary* symptoms by normal text type set in normal capitals and lower case.

If you are a Westerner, unfamiliar with Chinese medicine, you may find it helpful to refer back to the "A Brief Introduction to Chinese Medicine" in the first pages of this book before using these diagrams for your own self-diagnosis.

1

八味地黄丸

1. Pa-Wei-Ti-Huang-Wan
Rehmannia Eight Formula

Herb Ingredients: Rehmannia—8.0gm; Cornus—4.0gm; Poria (Hoelen)—3.0gm; Cinnamon—1.0gm; Dioscorea—4.0gm; Alisma—3.0gm; Moutan—3.0gm; Aconite—1.0gm.

Pharmacology: Rehmannia is a cardiotonic, diuretic, and hemostatic which has also been proven to lower blood sugar. Aconite is also a cardiotonic as well as an analgesic and stimulant. Cinnamon is a stimulant, analgesic, stomachic, and tonic (especially for the cardiovascular system). Cornus is an astringent tonic. Moutan acts as an emmenagogue and antipyretic, and it is effective for infections of the digestive tract. Hoelen is a sedative and diuretic. Alisma is a diuretic.

Objective of Treatment: Although it has many applications, this formula is most widely used to treat kidney disorders and diabetes and to prevent senility. The term "kidney failure" as defined by modern medicine is a syndrome in which there is a decrease of kidney function, a hormone imbalance, and general debility. Rehmannia Eight Formula has been known to prevent or arrest this general deterioration of the body processes, assuring a vigorous old age.

Physical Confirmation: Weak or mixed. Physical confirmation (body type) may be classified as either strong, weak, or mixed. Rehmannia Eight Formula is given to those of good complexion with obesity of the lower torso. (The term "obesity" means broadness, wideness, distension—not overweight.)

166

Symptoms: 1) Loss of vigor, low back pain, gradual loss of eyesight, and a tendency to become easily fatigued.

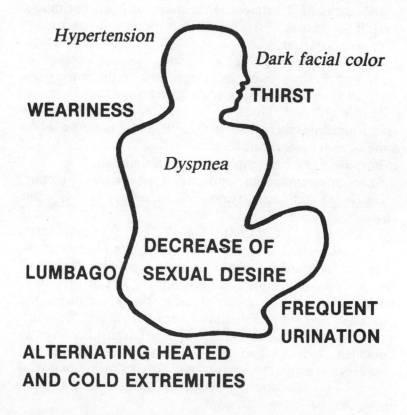

Hypertension

Dark facial color

THIRST

WEARINESS

Dyspnea

DECREASE OF
SEXUAL DESIRE

LUMBAGO

FREQUENT
URINATION

ALTERNATING HEATED
AND COLD EXTREMITIES

2

小柴胡湯

2. Hsiao-Chai-Hu-Tang
(Minor Bupleurum Combination)

Herbs Used: Bupleuri Radix, Pinelliae Rhizoma, Zingiberis Recens Rhizoma, Glycyrrhizae Radix, Scutellariae Radix, Ginseng Radix, Zizyphi Sativae Fructus

Objectives of Treatment: Bronchitis, asthma, peritonitis, tonsillitis, otitis media; and inflammations and neuroses of liver, gall, and stomach.

Physical Conditions: The moderate, muscular, and lady's types with flexible lower abdomen. Most of the patients are nervous, fond of cleanliness, and over laboring.

Modes of Fever: Moderate, light, and unidentified child-fever; and that alternating with chill, or is not receded by antibiotics or other substances.

Purpose: Principal symptoms: chest distention.

Subordinate symptoms: anorexia, heart distress, vomiting, excessive throat dryness, stomach ache, and fever with white coating on tongue.

Indications: (1) Cold with 3 to 5 day's fever, anorexia, cough and mucous sputum. (2) Acute or chronic bronchitis, asthma, peritonitis, and pneumonia. (3) Hepatitis, cholecystitis, gall stone, and jaundice. (4) Gastritis, sour stomach, decrease of acidity in stomach, peptic ulcer, and gastralgia. (5) Lymphadenitis, scrofula, tonsillitis, otitis media, mumps, and mastitis. (6) Pyelonephritis, fever in childbirth, and chill and fever due to uterine diseases. (7) Neuroses, stammer, epilepsy, male impotence, and oval alopecia. (8) Childhood mental instability and adenoid physique.

168

Note: For the strong physique with constipation and stomach, liver, and gall ailments—Major Bupleurum Combination.

NEUROTIC AILMENTS
(SENSITIVE)

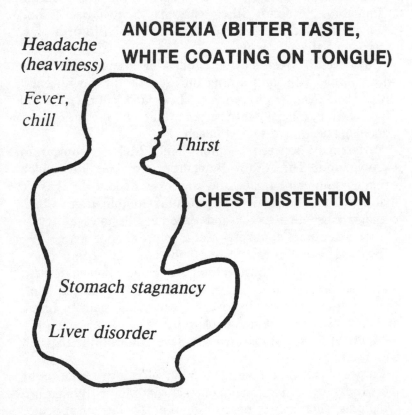

Headache (heaviness)

ANOREXIA (BITTER TASTE, WHITE COATING ON TONGUE)

Fever, chill

Thirst

CHEST DISTENTION

Stomach stagnancy

Liver disorder

3

大柴胡湯

3. Ta-Chai-Hu-Tang
(Major Bupleurum Combination)

Herbs Used: Bupleuri Radix, Pinelliae Rhizoma, Aurantii Immaturus Fructus, Rhei Rhizoma, Scutellariae Radix, Zingiberis Recens Rhizoma, Paeoniae Lactiflorae Radix, Zizyphy Sativae Fructus

Objectives of Treatment: The following complaints of those with a broad chin and strong muscles, or those with chest distress and average physique: (1) Liver and gall diseases. (2) Hypertension, partial deafness, and tinnitus. (3) Peptic ulcer, duodenum ulcer, and sour stomach.

Difference between Minor and Major Bupleurum Combination: The Minor Bupleurum Combination, which contains Ginseng, treats the anorexia caused by gastric malfunction. The Major Bupleurum Combination, which contains Aurantii Fructus and Paeonia, alleviates muscular tension and purges abnormal heat to improve appetite.

Physical Conditions: Strong muscles, fair complexion, broad face and chin, burly physique, strong lower abdomen, and fast defecation or constipation. Also indulged diet, chronic disease caused by over-fatigue, acute pain in fever, and nervousness of the strong physique.

Modes of Fever: Moderate fever, fever, and alternating chill with fever.

Purpose: This herb formula is mainly used for sensation of more obvious distention than that of Minor Bupleurum symptoms, such as: (1) chest distention, (2) loss of appetite,

(3) heart distention, (4) expiration, (5) abdominal distention, and (6) constipation.

Indications: (1) Liver malfunction, gall stone, and cholecystitis. (2) Hypertension, and mental instability. (3) Sour stomach, gastritis, peptic ulcer, duodenum ulcer, and tendency towards constipation. (4) Obeseness, stridor, shoulder stiffness due to difficult breathing, diabetes mellitus, apoplexia, tinnitus, and hearing retardation.

Note: For those suffering from diarrhea, a combination of equal amounts of Minor Bupleurum Combination and Hoelen 5 Herbs Formula should be prescribed.

HYPERTENSION

Heaviness of head

Insomnia

Tinnitus

YELLOW COATING ON TONGUE

Exhalation

CHEST DISTRESS

STOMACH STAGNANCY

LIVER DISTURBANCE

CONSTIPATION

柴胡桂枝湯

4. Chai-Hu-Kuei-Chih-Tang
(Bupleurum and Cinnamon Combination)

Herbs Used. Bupleuri Radix, Pinelliae Rhizoma, Zingiberis Recens Rhizoma, Paeoniae Lactiflorae Radix, Glycyrrhizae Radix, Scutellariae Radix, Ginseng Radix, Cinnamomi Ramulus, Zizyphi Sativae Fructus

Objectives of Treatment: Cold due to weak physique, stomach ache, peptic ulcer, hepatitis, cholecystitis, autonomic nervous irregularity, and metrorrhagia.

Pharmacology: This remedy is a compound prescription of Minor Bupleurum Combination and Cinnamon Combination. Burpleurum promotes the blood circulation of the liver, warms the trunk, and relieves chest distention and flushing heat. Scutellaria also has a heat relief action, especially in heat of the chest and inflammation of the digestive system. It will produce better results when used with Bupleurum. Ginseng strengthens the visceral functions and promotes the appetite. Zingiber and Pinellia, which check vomiting and cough but promote appetite, have diuretic action and can remove stagnant moisture in the stomach and chest. Cinnamon Combination adjusts autonomic nerves, and Cinnamon treats flushing-up and headache. Paeonia promotes the motion of digestive system. When used with Zizyphus, Zingiber, and Glycyrrhiza, it has a tonic action and checks perspiration.

Modes of Fever: Moderate and mild fever.

Purpose: This herb formula is to treat the similar symptoms of Minor Bupleurum Combination, especially ambiguous weak physical strength, stomach or periumbilical pain, limbs' weariness, and yawning.

Indications: (1) Colds (treatment and prevention). (2) Gastroptosis, hyperacidity or hypoacidity of stomach, peptic ulcer, duodenum ulcer, pancreatitis, liver malfunction, hepatitis, gall stone, cholecystitis, jaundice, heart distention, and anorexia. (3) Peritonitis, abdominal pain, stomach distention, constipation, and chronic appendicitis. (4) Female metrorrhagia, headache, vertigo, stiffness of shoulders, melancholia, weariness of limbs, lower abdominal distention, menstrual irregularity, and constipation. (5) Slender body, and weak digestive system. (6) Epilepsy, mental instability, and autonomic nerves irregularity.

Note: This herb formula is suitable for peptic ulcer, hepatitis, gall stone, and tendency towards constipation of the average or skinny physique. For those of the strong physique, Major Bupleurum Combination is recommended.

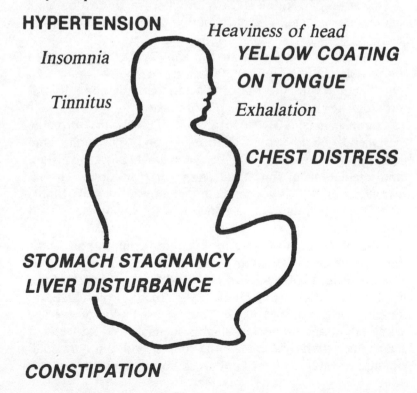

HYPERTENSION
Insomnia

Tinnitus

Heaviness of head

YELLOW COATING
ON TONGUE
Exhalation

CHEST DISTRESS

STOMACH STAGNANCY
LIVER DISTURBANCE

CONSTIPATION

5

人參當芍散

5. Jen-Sheng-Tang-Shao-San
(Ginseng and Tang-Kuei Formula)
Herbs Used: Ginseng Radix, Paeoniae Lactiflorae Radix, Atractylodis Alba Rhizoma, Alismatis Rhizoma, Glycyrrhizae Radix, Angelicae Sinensis Radix, Ligustici Wallichii Rhozoma, Poria (Hoelen), Cinnamomi Cortex
Objectives of Treatment: Soft muscles, fragile health, facial pallor, edema, chills, gynaecopathy, anemia, hemorrhoids, etc.
Purpose: This herb formula is mainly applied to strengthen blood circulation and metabolism of body fluids. In combination with the Major 4 Herbs Combination, it will promote the visceral function of both sexes.
Pharmacology: Glycyrrhiza and Ligusticum promote peripheral blood-vessel dilation, blood nutrition, and sedation. Paeonia has effects of analgesia, anti-convulsion, and regulation of intestinal vermicular motion. Alisma, Atractylodes, and Poria regulate metabolism of body fluids, and treat palpitation, dizziness, watery stomach, and rheumatism.
Note: Patients unsuitable to this herb formula should take the Bupleurum and Cinnamon Combination.
Diagnostic Findings: (Fragile health) (1) Slender face, fingers, and neck. (2) Skinny body, and narrow chest. (3) Fragile obeseness, and weak muscles. (4) Pallor or average complexion, and dryness of skin as anemia. (5) Cold feet and waist, but with hot face. (6) Fond of hot food, but only small amount of intake. (7) Low or weak voice, stammer, or high tone.

For those with skinny physique, edema, soft muscles, anemic complexion, chillphobia, and anorexia, this herb formula will promote blood circulation and improve vitality.

Note: (1) For those suffering from chills in lower trunk with flushing up, Cinnamon and Hoelen Formula may be administered. (2) For the purpose of beautifying the muscles, its combination with Coicis Semen may be used. To treat irregularities of autonomous nerves, a combination of equal amounts of this herb formula and Cinnamon and Hoelen Formula may be prescribed. (3) Women with chillphobia and habitual abortion got pregnant after taking this prescription in many cases.

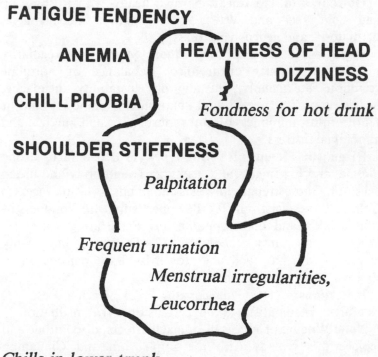

FATIGUE TENDENCY

ANEMIA   **HEAVINESS OF HEAD**
                           DIZZINESS

CHILLPHOBIA   *Fondness for hot drink*

SHOULDER STIFFNESS

Palpitation

Frequent urination

Menstrual irregularities,
Leucorrhea

Chills in lower trunk

6

桂枝茯苓丸

6. Kuei-Chih-Fu-Ling-Wan
(Cinnamon and Hoelen Formula)
Herbs Used: Cinnamomi Ramulus, Paeoniae Lactiflorae
Radix, Moutan Radicis Cortex, Poria (Hoelen), Persicae
Semem
Objectives of Treatment: Normal health with flushing up
and cold feet and waist; gynaecopathy, metrorrhagia,
dermatosis, and neuro-symptoms.
Symptoms of Extravasated Blood: Menstrual irregularity
may cause circular disturbance, imbalance of hormone
secretion, melancholy, flushing up, instability, headache,
heaviness of head, emotional abnormality, amnesia, cold or
febrile limbs, numbness of limbs, purple lips and gingiva, and
abdominal distress.
Diagnostic Findings: (Strong type) (1) Broad face, strong
muscle, and big fingers and neck. (2) Tough body and broad
chest. (3) Good strength in wrists and hands. (4) Pink face. (5)
Cold feet and waist, but febrile upper trunk. (6) Fondness of
cold drinks, and good appetite. (7) Penetrating voice. (8)
Mucous but scanty leucorrhea. (9) Dark red but scanty
menses, with a tendency towards late periods. (10)
Extravasated blood due to injury.
Indications: (1) Gynaecopathy, (2) Dermatoses, (3)
Neuralgia, rheumatism, and hypertension, (4) Constipation.
Note: When it produces ill stomach effects, discontinue and
replace this remedy with the Bupleurum and Cinnamon
Combination.

176

Note: Those with chillphobia and anemia should take Ginseng and Tang-Kuei Formula; for the purpose of beautifying muscles, its combination with Coicis Semen may be applied.

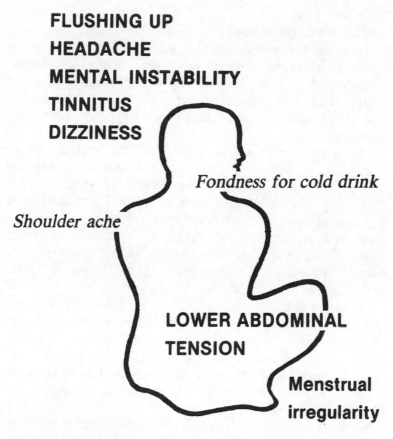

FLUSHING UP
HEADACHE
MENTAL INSTABILITY
TINNITUS
DIZZINESS

Fondness for cold drink

Shoulder ache

LOWER ABDOMINAL TENSION

Menstrual irregularity

Chills in lower trunk

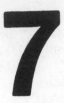

葛根湯

7. Ko-Ken-Tang
(Pueraria Combination)

Herbs Used: Puerariae Radix, Cinnamomi Cortex, Zizyphi Sativae Fructus, Glycyrrhizae Radix, Ephedrae Herba, Paeoniae Lactiflorae Radix, Zingiberis Recens Rhizoma

Objectives of Treatment: Primary cold, bad chill, headache, fever, stuffy nose, suppuration, stiffness of the shoulders, and neuralgia.

Pharmacology: Pueraria promotes the surface blood circulation of the body, relieves heat, and contracts the intestine for easy defecation. Ephedra in conjunction with Glycyrrhiza treat cough and warm the trunk. Ephedra when in conjunction with Cinnamon have perspiratory action. Cinnamon regulates blood circulation. Paeonia promotes digestic function and has tonic action. Glycyrrhiza detoxicates poisons in the liver. Zizyphus functions as glucose and folic acid. Zingiber helps blood circulation.

Purpose and Indications: (1) Colds. (2) Headache, and hot sensation with mucous diarrhea. (3) Stiffness of the shoulders, 40 years' wrist, 50 years' shoulders, stiffness of muscles, metrorrhagia, hypertension, and tendinitis. (4) Dermatoses, eczema, tinea, urticaria, measles, and local swelling with fever. (5) Ophthalmic diseases. (6) Ear and nose diseases. (7) Mental over-exertion.

Note: (1) When suffering from cold, take this herb formula with warm water and keep the body warm, will result in perspiration; repeat the same if perspiration does not occur in 2 or 3 hours. (2) For those with mild fatigue after perspiration, tendency towards cold, and gastrointestinal feebleness; the Bupleurum and Cinnamon Combination should be prescribed for the first symptoms.

Indications: (1) Primary cold, bad chill, headache, no perspiration, mild cough, shoulder stiffness, 40 years' wrists, 50 years' shoulders, and stuffy nose. (2) Cold with diarrhea, acute enteritis, mucous stools, urticaria, conjunctivitis, and keratitis.

NO PERSPIRATION

HEADACHE

Stuffy nose

NECK STIFFNESS   *Fever, bad chill*

SHOULDER STIFFNESS

TENSENESS OF

NECK AND BACK

Diarrhea

8

五苓散

8. Wu-Ling-San
Hoelen Five Herbs Formula

Herb Ingredients: Polyporus—4.5gm; Atractylodes—4.5gm; Cinnamon—3.0gm; Poria (Hoelen)—6.5gm; Alisma—6.0gm.

Pharmacology: Although the individual herbs in this formula are not particularly effective alone as diuretics, together they produce diuresis whenever there is edema. This effect does not occur in healthy persons, only in those whose fluid metabolism is out of balance.

Objectives of Treatment: This formula is effective for any condition in which there is an excess of or an imbalance in the body fluids.

Physical Confirmation: Mixed.

Symptoms: 1) Thirst accompanied by perspiration and dysuria. 2) Fever, dysuria, thirst, and vomiting after drinking water. 3) Vomiting, diarrhea, thirst, dysuria, and generalized pain. 4) Thirst, obiguria, and edema. 5) Edema.

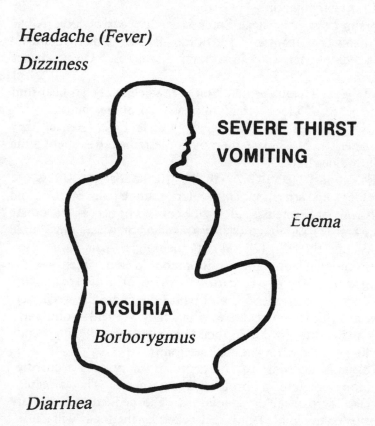

Headache (Fever)
Dizziness

SEVERE THIRST
VOMITING

Edema

DYSURIA
Borborygmus

Diarrhea

9

薏苡仁湯

9. I-Yi-Jen-Tang
(Coix Combination)

Herbs Used: Angelicae Sinensis Radix, Atractylodis Alba Rhizoma, Paeoniae Lactiflorae Radix, Coicis Semen, Ephedrae Herba, Cinnamomi Ramulus, Glycyrrhizae Radix.

Analgesic Treatment of Chinese Medicine: (1) To heal the disturbance of blood circulation; (2) To purge the moist in joints or tissues; (3) To relieve muscle tone. Hence, the characteristic of Chinese therapy is the radical treatment and without side effects.

Indications: Neuralgia, arthritis, rheumatism, stiffness of shoulders, and sensational muscular or numb pain.

Neuralgia: Severe pain along the courses of nerves, the most cases are: (1) Lumbago (sciatica)—pains at waist, hips, and back of thighs. (2) Wrist neuralgia—pain due to inconventional labor, and outdoor labor in cold winter.

Arthritis: (1) Wrist arthritis—wrist arthritis over 40, shoulder stiffness over 50, and pain in bending the wrist. (2) Knee arthritis (often occurs in climacteric women)—mild pain in walking but severe in bending and straightening, and swelling or even edema at the knee joints.

Rheumatism: Most of the acute, primary, and recurring symptoms require a prolonged treatment. The affected muscles are painful or edematous. The deductive muscular arthritis or the joints being reattacked by the focus will cause fever.

Note: For common neuralgia, arthritis, rheumatism, chills in lower trunk, and anemia, Cinnamon and Atractylodes Combination or a combination of equal amounts of this herb formula and Ginseng and Tang-Kuei Formula should be prescribed. For additional internal bleeding due to wounds, Cinnamon and Hoelen Formula should be taken at first so as to remove the extravasated blood.

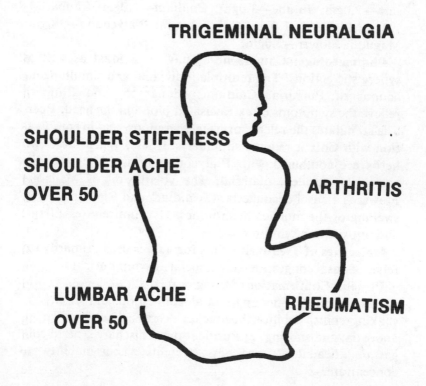

TRIGEMINAL NEURALGIA

SHOULDER STIFFNESS
SHOULDER ACHE
OVER 50

ARTHRITIS

LUMBAR ACHE
OVER 50

RHEUMATISM

10

清鼻湯

10. Ching-Pi-Tang
Pueraria Nasal Combination

Herb Ingredients: Pueraria—4.0gm; Ma-Huang—4.0gm; Cinnamon—2.0gm; Paeonia—2.0gm; Ginger—1.0gm; Gypsum—2.0gm; Jujube—3.0gm; Cnidium—2.0gm; Rhubarb—1.0gm; Licorice—1.0gm; Coix—3.0gm; Platycodon—3.0gm; Magnolia Flower—2.0gm.

Pharmacology: Chinese herbs have individual as well as synergistic actions. The multiple individual and simultaneous actions of Pueraria, Cnidium, Cinnamon, and Rhubarb relieve the symptoms of extravasated blood in the head. Pueraria stimulates the release of nasal secretions, and in combination with Coix it relieves shoulder stiffness. When these two herbs are combined with Platycodon bring about the discharge of purulent material. The volatile oil of Magnolia Flower is a nasal decongestant. Cnidium and Rhubarb relieve swelling of the mucous membranes. Gypsum relieves allergic and intoxication symptoms.

Objectives of Treatment: This formula is used primarily for relief of nasal congestion and associated symptoms.

Physical Confirmation: Strong or mixed.

Symptoms: 1) Sneezing, nasal congestion and discharge, shaking chills, debility, headache, decreased sense of smell, anorexia, and snoring. 2) Purulent nasal discharge, nasal congestion, headache, weakness, debility, and inability to concentrate.

Indications: The following disorders are considered to be part of the Pueraria Nasal Combination confirmation: 1) Rhinitis (symptom set #1)—acute and chronic. This formula has been particularly effective in bringing about total relief from chronic rhinitis. 2) Sinusitis (symptom set #2)—acute and chronic.

Early treatment produces good results in acute cases; chronic cases are more difficult to cure. Surgery may be effective; but it is sometimes necessary to repeat the procedure, and the postoperative care is difficult and prolonged. Prompt treatment with this formula can prevent the necessity of more radical treatment.

Contraindications: None.

Alternate Formulas: Allergy-induced rhinitis in which there is sneezing is treated with the Blue Dragon Combination.

HEADACHE

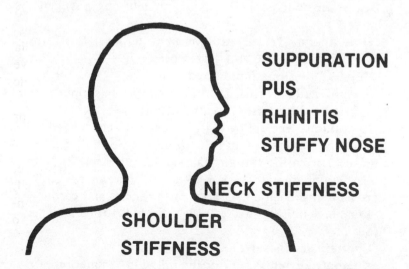

SUPPURATION
PUS
RHINITIS
STUFFY NOSE
NECK STIFFNESS
SHOULDER STIFFNESS

11

十味敗毒散

11. Shih-Wei-Pai-Tu-San
Bupleurum and Schizonepeta Formula

Herb Ingredients: Bupleurum—3.0gm; Siler—2.0gm; Cherry Bark—3.0gm; Ginger—1.0gm; Schizonepeta—1.0gm; Platycodon—3.0gm; Cnidium—3.0gm; Poria— (Hoelen)— 3.0gm; Tuhuo—2.0gm; Licorice—1.0gm.

Pharmacology: This formula was first modified by Kakou Seichiu, a well-known Japanese surgeon, according to his clinical experience. S. Asata later added to the formulation Forsythia, an herb whose antiphlogistic properties made this combination an excellent dermatologic remedy. Recently, Dr. T. Yakaju, an accepted authority on Chinese medicine, stated that when Coix was added to this formula it would be more effective in nourishing the skin and relieving purulent discharge.

Objectives of Treatment: The main uses for this formula are chronic dermatitus and dermatoses.

Physical Confirmation: Mixed.

Symptoms: 1) Pruritis. 2) Inflammation and suppuration of skin lesions. 3) Blisters. 4) Lymphadenitis. 5) Mastitis.

Indications: The following disorders are considered to be part of the Bupleurum and Schizonepeta Formula confirmation: 1) Dermatitis (inflammatory skin disease). 2) Dermatoses (noninflammatory skin disease)—acute or subacute. 3) Eczema and subacute urticaria. 4) Furuncles and carbuncles. 5) Lymphadenitis. 6) Boils. 7) Mastitis. 8) Scrofula and "scald head".

Contraindications: None.

Alternate Formulas: 1) For the initial inflammation of skin diseases, Pueraria Combination is given for the first two or three days; then this formula is prescribed. 2) Those with allergies and an average constitution can develop a strong constitution by taking equal amounts of this formula and Minor Bupleurum Combination over a long period of time.

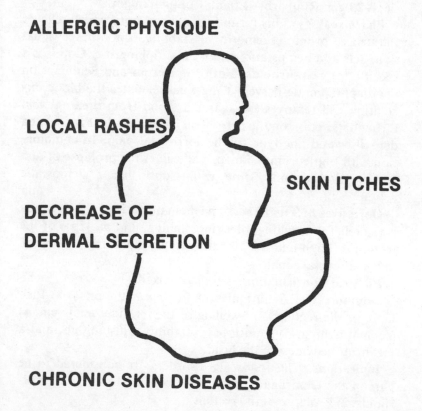

ALLERGIC PHYSIQUE

LOCAL RASHES

SKIN ITCHES

DECREASE OF
DERMAL SECRETION

CHRONIC SKIN DISEASES

12

乙字湯

12. I-Tzu-Tang

Cimifuga Combination

Herb Ingredients: Bupleurum—5.0gm; Tang-Kuei—6.0gm; Cimifuga—1.5gm; Jujube—1.2gm; Scute—3.0gm; Licorice—2.0gm; Rhubarb—1.0gm; Coptis—2.0gm.

Pharmacology: This formula contains Coptis which relieves flatulence, promotes emotional stability, smoothes evacuation, acts as a hemostatic, and is an antiphlogistic. Coptis is a specific for hemorrhoids. Both Bupleurum and Scute act on the diaphragmatic nerves. Tang-Kuei regulates the blood circulation and removes extravasated blood from the anal vein through its action on the peripheral blood vessels. Licorice is a detoxifier and anodyne for hemorrhoidal pain. In combination with Bupleurum, Cimifuga alleviates the prolapse of and retracts the rectum. Scute with Coptis has a hemostatic action.

Objectives of Treatment: The main purpose of this formula is the relief of swelling, bleeding, itching, and prolapse of the rectum through removal of extravasated blood from the veins in the anorectal canal.

Physical Confirmation: Strong or mixed.

Symptoms: 1) Aching and/or itching at the anus. 2) Prolapse of the rectum. 3) Swelling of the terminal anal vein. 4) Vaginal itching. 5) Emotional instability, flushing-up, and a feeling of heaviness in the head.

Indications: The following disorders are considered to be part of the Cimifuga Combination confirmation: 1) Hemorrhoids. 2) Prolapse of the rectum.

Contraindications: None.

Alternate Formulas: 1) Those of weak confirmation with the above symptoms are given Cinnamon and Paeonia Combination instead. 2) If diarrhea occurs with use of this formula, Ginseng and Tang-Kuei Formula is given as a replacement. 3) For women with a tendency towrds flushing up, Cinnamon and Hoelen Combination should be given instead. 4) If there is severe constipation, Coptis and Rhubarb Combination should be taken before sleep. 5) Lithospermum Ointment is very effective when applied externally.

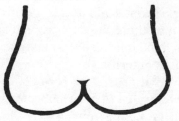

Hemorrhoidal bleeding   **BLIND PILES**

Prolapse of rectum

CONSTIPATION

ACUTE PAIN

189

13

三黃錠

13. San-Huang-Ting
Coptis and Rhubarb Combination

Herb Ingredients: Rhubarb—2.0gm; Scute—1.0gm; Coptis—1.0gm.

Pharmacology: Rhubarb is a cathartic. In combination with Scute and Coptis, it provides relief for gout and acts as an antiphlogistic and decongestant. Scute and Coptis act together as a stomachic and for relief of chest distress due to cardiac disorders. Coptis alone has hemostatic action. The synergistic action of these three herbs regulates bile secretion, has a laxative action, relieves inflammation with congestion, and alleviates gastroenteritis.

Objectives of Treatment: This formula is used to treat disorders and symptoms due to or complicated by constipation.

Physical Confirmation: Strong.

Symptoms: 1) Habitual constipation. 2) Flushing-up, facial flushing, emotional instability, tinnitus, a feeling of heaviness in the head, shoulder stiffness. 3) Hypertension. 4) Hemorrhoidal bleeding. 5) Epistaxis.

Indications: The following disorders are considered to be part of the Coptis and Rhubarb Combination confirmation: 1) Habitual constipation. 2) Stomach distress and gastrorrhagia. 3) Hypertension. 4) Arteriosclerosis. 5) Liver diseases. 6) Stroke (treatment and prevention). 7) Hemorrhoids. 8) Epistaxis.

HYPERTENSION

**MENTAL INSTABILITY
(HOT TEMPER)**

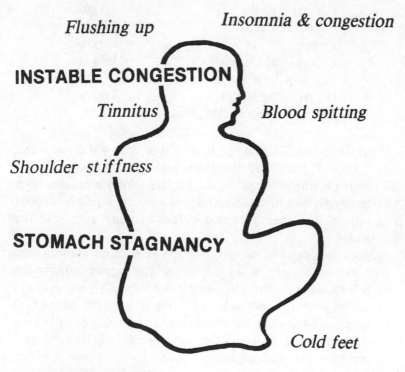

Flushing up   *Insomnia & congestion*

INSTABLE CONGESTION

Tinnitus   *Blood spitting*

Shoulder stiffness

STOMACH STAGNANCY

Cold feet

**CONSTIPATION
(WITH BLEEDING)**

THE APPLICATION AND DOSAGE OF CHINESE HERB FORMULAS

Chinese herb formulas were decocted for application until recent time. The herbs required were placed together with water, decocted and boiled over a weak fire, and then applied with dregs removed. Take Ko-Ken-Tang 葛根湯 Pueraria Combination) for example, the components of this formula are as follows:

Puerariae Radix	8.0 gm.
Ephedrae Herba	4.0 gm.
Zizyphi Sativae Fructus	4.0 gm.
Cinnamomi Cortex	3.0 gm.
Paeoniae Lactiflorae Radix	3.0 gm.
Glycyrrhizae Radix	2.0 gm.
Zingiberis Recens Rhizoma	1.0 gm.

Pueraria and Ma Huang are first cooked with 400 cc. of water over a low fire until 80 cc. of the water has evaporated. The white foam which forms on the surface is removed, the other herbs added, and formula simmered until the liquid is reduced to 120 cc. It is then decanted before administering it to the patient.

Since this method of preparation is time-consuming and inconvenient, many Asian countries have begun refining the herb formulas into granules and powders using precise apparatus and scientific methods. This pre-preparation of the formulas allows for their availability and convenience of use by the patient; it also prevents loss of some of the effective ingredients through inaccuracy of preparation in the the old method.

The dosage of these scientifically prepared Chinese formulas is 4.5 to 6.0 gm. to be divided in three equal doses each day. That is, 1.5 to 2.0 gm. is to be taken with lukewarm water three times a day either between or just after meals.

Occasionally, the addition of other herbs to the basic formula is necessary. In this case, two-thirds of the original formula is taken while each new herb is added in the amount of one-third of the original quantity. For example, if the daily dosage of Ko-Ken-Tang is 4.0 gm. and Chuan-Chiung (Cnidium) and Hsin-I (Magnolia Flower) are to be added, these two herbs would be added in the amount of 1.0 gm. each.

THE TOXICITY OF
CHINESE HERB FORMULAS

Although Western medicines are effective for some diseases, they do have side effects. Because of their toxicity, the frequent use of many Western medicines can be harmful to the body.

By contrast, the toxicity of Chinese herb formulas is very low. The author studied the toxicities of three hundred different Chinese herb formulas and found this to be impressively true.

For example: with toxicity expressed as LD_{50}, a man weighing 60 kilograms (roughly 150 pounds) would have to ingest somewhere between 120 and 300 grams of a typical formula to reach LD_{50} and endanger his life. Since the Chinese dosages are never more than a few grams, this is manifestly impossible.

Thus, their low toxicity is one reason Chinese herb formulas will long exist.

WHERE YOU CAN BUY CHINESE HERB FORMULAS

Worldwide, over one billion people use Chinese herb formulas, and herb shops are ubiquitous throughout Hong Kong, Singapore, Korea, Japan, and China. It has been estimated that, in Taiwan alone, there are over 8,000 herbal apothecaries.

Though almost all the prescriptions presented in this book are available in Chinese herb stores in the United States, they must be decocted at home before use. In order to make treatment with Chinese herbs more convenient and thereby more acceptable to Western patients, the author pioneered and perfected the manufacturing of concentrated herbal granules. For 40 years, the Sun Ten Pharmaceutical Works Co., Ltd., which was founded by Dr. Hong-yen Hsu, has been a leader in the processing of scientifically prepared, convenient, and effective herb products.

As the most prestigious supplier of Chinese herb formulas in Asia, Sun Ten's line of quality products may be ordered through the following distributors:

WEST COAST
Brion Herbs Corp. 9250 Jeronimo Rd. Irvine, CA 92718
(714) 587-1238 Phone   (800) 333-HERB Orders
(714) 587-1260 Fax   (800) 777-2309 Consultation

EUROPE
Biomed. Hoevenstraat 45, 2160 Wommelgem, Belgium
(03) 354-0333 Phone   (03) 354-0377 Fax

APPENDIX OF HERBS AND THEIR USES

Chinese Name (Transliteration)	Common Name	Part Used	Scientific Name (Family Name)	Medical Uses
冬 葵 子 (Tung-kuei-tzu)	Abutilon	Seed	*Abutilon avicennae* Gaertn. (Malvaceae)	Demulcent, smooth the intestine, diuretic, stomachic
五 加 皮 (Wu-chia-pi)	Acanthopanax	Root epidermis	*Acanthopanax gracilistylus* W. W. Smith (Araliaceae)	Antirheumatism, sexual potency, restoring vigor
牛 膝 (Niu-hsi)	Achyranthes	Root	*Achyranthes bidentata* Blume (Amaranthaceae)	Diuretic, emmenagogue, mucilaginous, demulcent

Chinese Name (Transliteration)	Common Name	Part Used	Scientific Name (Family Name)	Medical Uses
附 子 (Fu-tzu)	Aconite	Root	*Aconitum carmichaeli* Debx. (Ranunculaceae)	Stimulant, cardio-tonic, analgesic
石 菖 蒲 (Shih-chang-pu)	Acorus	Rhizome	*Acorus gramineus* Soland. (Araceae)	Stomachic in dispepsia, hyperacidity
陽 起 石 (Yang-chi-shih)	Actinolite	Mineral	Calcium and Magnesium Silicates	Tonic and antispasmodic in colic, prostatitis, amenorrhea.
南 沙 參 (Nan-sha-sheng)	Adenophora	Root	*Adenophora verticillata* Fisch.; *A. stricta* Miq. (Campanulaceae)	Expectorant, sialagogue
藿 香 (Huo-shiang)	Agastache	Herb	*Agastache rugosa* O. Kuntze (Labiatae)	Carminative, stomachic

Chinese Name (Transliteration)	Common Name	Part Used	Scientific Name (Family Name)	Medical Uses
白 花 蛇 (Pai-hua-sheh)	Agkistrodon	Body	*Agkistrodon acutus* Guenther (Gotalidae)	Antisyphilitic, anthelmintic
仙 鶴 草 (龍芽草) (Hsien-ho-tsao)	Agrimony	Herb	*Agrimonia pilosa* Ledeb. *A. eupatoria* L. (Rosaceae)	Astringent hemostatic in enterorrhagia, hematuria; cardiotonic
木 通 (Mu-tung)	Akebia	Stem	*Akebia quinata* Decne; (Ranunculaceae) *Clematis armandi* Franch. (Lardizabalaceae)	Diuretic, antiphlogistic
澤 瀉 (Tse-hsieh)	Alisma	Tuber	*Alisma plantago* L. (Alismataceae)	Diuretic, diaphoretic

Chinese Name (Transliteration)	Common Name	Part Used	Scientific Name (Family Name)	Medical Uses
葱 白 (Chung-pai)	Allium	Bulb	*Allium fistulosun* (Liliaceae)	Stomachic, diuretic, anthelmintic
蘆 薈 (Lu-huei)	Aloe	Leaves juice	*Aloe vera* L. (Liliaceae)	Laxative, stomachic, emmenagogue
九 節 菖 蒲 (Chiu-chieh-chang-pu)	Altaica	Rhizome	*Anemone altaica* Fisch. (Ranunculaceae)	Stimulant, expectorant, detoxifier
明 礬 (Ming-fan)	Alum	Mineral	$KAl_3(SO_4)_2 \cdot 12H_2O$	Astringent, hemostatic, anthelmintic, detoxifier
白 蘞 (Pai-lien)	Ampelopsis	Root	*Ampelopsis japonica* (Thunb.) Makino (Vitaceae)	Antipyretic, detoxifier, nourish the muscle, analgesic

Chinese Name (Transliteration)	Common Name	Part Used	Scientific Name (Family Name)	Medical Uses
知 母 (Chih-mu)	Anemarrhena	Rhizome	*Anemarrhena asphodeloides* Bunge. (Liliaceae)	Antipyretic, expectorant
白 頭 翁 (Pai-tou-weng)	Anemone	Root	*Anemone cernua* Thunb., *A. pulsatilla* (Ranunculaceae)	Antidiarrheic
白 芷 (Pai-chih)	Angelica	Root	*Angelica dahurica* var. *pai-chi; Angelica dahurica* Benth.et Hook. (Umbelliferae)	Aromatic, stimulant, analgesic
穿 山 甲 (Chuan-shan-chia)	Anteater Scales	Scales	*Manis pentadactyla* L. (Manidae)	Stimulate the circulation, dispel the pus

Chinese Name (Transliteration)	Common Name	Part Used	Scientific Name (Family Name)	Medical Uses
羚 羊 角 (Ling-yang-chueh)	Antelope Horn	Horn	*Saiga tatarica* L. *Nemorhaedus cripus* (Bovidae)	Antispasmodic, antipyretic, tonic
杏 仁 (Hsing-jen)	Apricot Seed (Almond)	Seed	*Prunus armeniaca* L. (Rosaceae)	Antitussive, sedative in bronchitis, asthma
沈 香 (Shen-shiang)	Aquilaria	Wood	*Aquilaria agallocha* Roxb. (Thymelaeaceae)	Stomachic in gastralgia, colic, nervous emesis
牛 蒡 子 (Niu-pang-tzu)	Arctium	Fruit	*Arctium lappa* L. (Compositae)	Diuretic, antipyretic, expectorant, antiphlogistic

Chinese Name (Transliteration)	Common Name	Part Used	Scientific Name (Family Name)	Medical Uses
大 腹 皮 (Ta-fu-pi)	Areca	Fruit rind	*Areca catechu* L. (Palmae)	Diuretic
檳 榔 (Pin-lang)	Areca Seed	Seed	*Areca catechu* L. (Palmae)	Astringent, taeniafuga
天 南 星 (Tien-nan-hsing)	Arisaema	Tuber	*Arisaema amurense* Maximowicz (Araceae)	Analgesic, antis- pasmodic, taeniafuge
馬 兜 鈴 (Ma-tou-ling)	Aristolochia	Fruit	*Aristolochia contorta* Bunge; *A. debilis* Sieb. et Zucc. (Aristolochiaceae)	Expectorant, antitussive
艾 葉 (Ai-yeh)	Artemisia (Mugwort)	Leaves	*Artemisia vulgaris* L. (Compositae)	Hemostatic, stomachic

Chinese Name (Transliteration)	Common Name	Part Used	Scientific Name (Family Name)	Medical Uses
阿魏 (Ah-wei)	Asafoetida	Gum-resin	*Ferula assafoetida* (L.) (Umbelliferae)	Vermicide, sedative, antispasmodic, digestive
細辛 (Hsi-hsin)	Asarum	Herb	*Asarum sieboldi* Miq. (Aristolochiaceae)	Analgesic, sedative, expectorant
天門冬 (Tien-men-tong)	Asparagus	Root	*Asparagus cochinchinensis* Merr. (Liliaceae)	Diuretic, expectorant
紫菀 (Tzu-wan)	Aster	Root	*Aster tartaricus* L.f. (Compositae)	Antitussive, expectorant
黃耆 (Huang-chi)	Astragalus	Root	*Astragalus hoantchy* Franchet (Leguminosae)	Tonic, diuretic, antipyretic

Chinese Name (Transliteration)	Common Name	Part Used	Scientific Name (Family Name)	Medical Uses
白 朮 (Pai-chu)	Atractylodes (White Atractylodes)	Rhizome	*Atractylodes ovata* DC. *A. macrocephala* Koidz. (Compositae)	Aromatic, tonic, chronic gastro-enteritis
蒼 朮 (Tsang-chu)	Atractylodes	Rhizome	*Atractylodes ovata* DC. *A. lancea* DC. (Compositae)	Aromatic, tonic, chronic gastroenteritis
橘 皮 (Chu-pi)	Aurantium	Fruit rind	*Citrus aurantium* L. (Rutaceae)	Stomachic, diges-tant, diaphoretic, expectorant, anti-tussive, antiemetic
薤 白 (Hsieh-pai)	Bakeri	Bulbus	*Allium bakeri* Regel, *A. macrostemon* Bge. (Liliaceae)	Smooth the "chi"

203

Chinese Name (Transliteration)	Common Name	Part Used	Scientific Name (Family Name)	Medical Uses
竹 茹 (Chu-ju)	Bamboo	Stem with outside skin removed	*Phyllostachys nigra* Munro (Gramineae)	Refrigerant, antipyretic, antitussive
竹 葉 (Chu-yeh)	Bamboo Leaves	Leaves	*Phyllostachys bambusoide* S. et Z. (Gramineae)	Antipyretic
竹 瀝 (Chu-li)	Bamboo Sap	Sap	*Phyllostachys nigra* Munro (Gramineae)	Expectorant, Antitussive
熊 膽 (Hsiung-tan)	Bear Gall	Gall	*Ursus arctos* L. (Ursidae)	Antiphlogistic, antipyretic, analgesic, antispasmodic
射 干 She-Kan	Belamcanda	Rhizome	*Belamcanda chinensis* (L.) DC. (Iridaceae)	Expectorant, antipyretic, stomachic, purgative

204

Chinese Name (Transliteration)	Common Name	Part Used	Scientific Name (Family Name)	Medical Uses
冬 瓜 子 (Tung-kua-tzu)	Benincasa	Seed	*Benincasa hispida* Cogn. *B. cerifera* Savi. (Cucurbitaceae)	Diuretic
安 息 香 (An-hsi-shiang)	Benzoin	Resin	*Styrax benzoin* Dryander *S. tonkinensis* Craib. (Styracaceae)	Expectorant, diuretic, bactericide
柏 子 仁 (Po-tzu-jen)	Biota	Seed	*Biota orientalis* (L.) Endl. (Cupressaceae)	Tonic, sedative, lenitive
青 木 香 (Ching-mu-shiang)	Birthwort	Root	*Aristolochia contorta* Bunge.(Aristolochiaceae)	Sedative
益 智 (I-chih)	Black Cardamon	Seed	*Elettaria cardamomum* Maton (Zingiberaceae)	Stomachic, tonic in gastralgia, enuresis, spermatorrhea

Chinese Name (Transliteration)	Common Name	Part Used	Scientific Name (Family Name)	Medical Uses
白 及 (Pai-chi)	Bletilla	Rhizome	*Bletilla striata* (Thunb.) Reichb. f. (Orchidaceae)	Nourish the muscle, hemostatic,
菁 皮 (Ching-pi)	Blue Citrus Peel	Fruit rind	*Citrus medica* L. (Rutaceae)	Aromatic, stomachic
冰 片 (Ping-pien)	Borneol	Crystal	*Dryobalanops aromatica* Gaertn.; *D. camphora* Colebr.(Dypterocarpaceae)	Antiphlogistic, antispasmodic, sedative, antitussive
牛 黃 (Niu-huang)	Bos	Calculus	*Bos taurus* var. *domestica* Gmelin (Bovidae)	Antitoxin, cardiotonic, antipyretic, sedative, diuretic
白 芥 子 (Pai-chieh-tzu)	Brassica	Seed	*Brassica alba* L. (Crucifereae)	Emetic

Chinese Name (Transliteration)	Common Name	Part Used	Scientific Name (Family Name)	Medical Uses
楮 實 子 (Chu-shih-tzu)	Broussonetia	Fruit	*Broussonetia papyrifera* Vent. (Moraceae)	Stimulant, diuretic, ophthalmic
鴉 膽 子 (Ya-tan-tzu)	Brucea	Seeds	*Brucea javanica* Merr. (Simarubaceae)	Anthelmintic
密 蒙 花 (Mi-meng-hua)	Buddleia	Flower	*Buddleia officinalis* Max. (Longaniaceae)	Ophthalmic in nyctalopia, asthenopia, cataract
蒲 黃 (Pu-huang)	Bulrush	Pollen	*Typha angustata* Bory et Chaub; *T. latifolia* L. (Typhaceae)	Hemostatic, diuretic, astringent, dessicant vulnerary
柴 胡 (Chai-hu)	Bupleurum	Root	*Bupleurum chinense* DC.*B. falcatum* L. (Umbelliferae)	Antipyretic, infunctional amenorrhea

Chinese Name (Transliteration)	Common Name	Part Used	Scientific Name (Family Name)	Medical Uses
血 竭 (Hsueh-chieh)	Calamus Gum	Resinous secretion	*Calamus draco* Willdenow (*Daemonorops draco* Blume) (Palmae)	Astringent, hemostatic, analgesic
寒 水 石 (Han-sui-shih)	Calcite	Mineral	$CaCO_3$	Antipyretic
輕 粉 (Ching-fen)	Calomel	Mineral	Hg_2Cl_2	Anthelmintic, digestic, diuretic, cathartic
火 麻 仁 (Huo-ma-jen)	Cannabis Seed	Seed	*Cannabis sativa* L. (Cannabiaceae)	Tonic, emollient
茵 陳 (Yin-chen)	Capillaris	Herb	*Artemisia capillaris* Thunb. (Compositae)	Diuretic, antipyretic in icterus

208

Chinese Name (Transliteration)	Common Name	Part Used	Scientific Name (Family Name)	Medical Uses
砂 仁 （ 縮 砂 ） (Sa-jen)	Cardamon	Fruit	*Amomum xanthioides* Wall.; *Hedychium coronarium* Koen. (Zingiberaceae)	Aromatic, stomachic, carminative
紅 花 (Hung-hua)	Carthamus	Flower	*Carthamus tinctorius* L. (Compositae)	Uterine astringent in dysmenorrhea
決 明 子 (Chueh-ming-tzu)	Cassia Seed	Seed	*Cassia tora* L. (Leguminosae)	Various eye and hepatic disorders
兒 茶 （ 阿仙藥 ） (Erh-cha)	Catechu	Resin	*Acacia catechu* (L.) Willd. (Leguminosae)	Astringent, refrigerant, antidiarrhea
青 葙 子 (Ching-hsiang-tzu)	Celosia	Seed	*Celosia argentea* L. (Amaranthaceae)	Ophthalmic

209

Chinese Name (Transliteration)	Common Name	Part Used	Scientific Name (Family Name)	Medical Uses
鹿茸 (Lu-jung)	Cervus	Velvet horn	*Cervus nippon* Temminck; *C. elaphus* L. (Cervidae)	Tonic, stimulant
鹿角 (Lu-chueh)	Cervus Horn	Horn	*Cervus nippon* Temminck; *C. elaphus* L. (Cervidae)	Dispel the effused blood, improve the circulation
鹿角膠 (Lu-chueh-chiao)	Cervus Colloid	Cervus horn processed by long cooking	*Cervus nippon* Temminck; (Cervidae)	Nutrient, nourish the liver and kidney
鉛粉 (Chien-fen)	Ceruse	Mineral	$2PbCO_3 \cdot Pb(OH)_2$	Anti-diarrhea, external use for ulcer

Chinese Name (Transliteration)	Common Name	Part Used	Scientific Name (Family Name)	Medical Uses
木 瓜 (Mu-kua)	Chaenomeles	Fruit	*Chaenomeles lagenaria* Koidz. (Rosaceae)	Astringent in diarrhea, analgesic in arthralgia, gout, cholera
櫻 皮 (Ying-pi)	Cherry Bark	Bark	*Prunus yedoensis* Matsumura (Rosaceae)	Astringent, antitussive
枳 殼 (Chih-ko)	Chih-Ko	Ripe fruit	*Citrus kotokan* (Rutaceae)	Excessive sputum, visceral, distention abdominal swelling
枳 實 (Chih-shih)	Chih-Shih	Unripe fruit	*Poncirus trifoliata* Rafin. (Rutaceae)	Stomachic for dysentery, tenesmus, antidiarrheic

Chinese Name (Transliteration)	Common Name	Part Used	Scientific Name (Family Name)	Medical Uses
秦 艽 (Chin-chiu)	Chin-Chiu	Root	*Gentiana macrophylla* Pall. (Gentianaceae)	Antipyretic, diuretic, exsiccant
青 礞 石 (Ching-meng-shih)	Chlorite	Mineral	Micaceous earth (A Silicate of Iron, Magnesium, and Aluminum)	Expectorant, digestive, antispasmodic
菊 花 (Chu-hua)	Chrysanthemum	Flower	*Chrysanthemum morifolium; C. indicum* (Compositae)	Sedative, refrigerant in headache, influenza
蟬 蛻 (Chan-shui)	Cicada	Exuviae	*Cryptotympana atrata* Fabr. (Cicadidae)	Antipyretic

Chinese Name (Transliteration)	Common Name	Part Used	Scientific Name (Family Name)	Medical Uses
升 麻 (Sheng-ma)	Cimicifuga	Root	*Cimicifuga dahurica* Maxim. *C. foetida* L. (Ranunculaceae)	Antipyretic, sedative, analgesic
硃 砂 (Chu-sha)	Cinnabar	Mineral	Red Mercuric sulfide	Antispasmodic, sedative in nervous tachycardia, infantile convulsions
桂 枝 (Kuei-chih)	Cinnamon	Ramulus	*Cinnamomum cassia* Blume (Lauraceae)	Aromatic, stomachic
桂 皮 (Kuei-pi)	Cinnamon	Bark	*Cinnamomum cassia* Blume (Lauraceae)	Astringent, tonic, analgesic, stimulant

Chinese Name (Transliteration)	Common Name	Part Used	Scientific Name (Family Name)	Medical Uses
肉 苁 蓉 (Jou-tsung-jung)	Cistanche	Herb	*Cistanche salsa* Benthament et Hooker (Orobanchaceae)	Aphrodisiac, tonic in spermatorrhea, impotence
陳 皮 (Chen-pi)	Citrus	Fruit rind	*Citrus nobilis* Lunr. (Rutaceae)	Stomachic, digestant, expectorant, antitussive, anthelmintic
威 靈 仙 (Wei-ling-hsien)	Clematis	Root	*Clematis chinensis* Osbeck (Ranunculaceae)	Analgesic, rheumatism, antipyretic, diuretic
臭 梧 桐 (Tso-wu-tung)	Clerodendron	Leaves	*Clerodendron trichotomum* Thunb. (Verbenaceae)	Hypotensor, sedative

Chinese Name (Transliteration)	Common Name	Part Used	Scientific Name (Family Name)	Medical Uses
丁 香 (Ting-shiang)	Clove	Flower	*Eugenia caryophyllata* Thunb. (Myrtaceae)	Aromatic, carminative, antiemetic, aromatic, stomachic
白 豆 蔻 (Pai-tou-kou)	Cluster	Fruit	*Amomum cardamomum* L. (Zingiberaceae)	Aromatic, stomachic with antiemetic action
川 芎 (Chuan-chiung)	Cnidium	Rhizome	*Cnidium officinale* Makino; *Ligusticum wallichii* Franch. (Umbelliferae)	Sedative, analgesic, emmenagogue
薏 苡 仁 (I-yi-jen)	Coix	Seed	*Coix lachryma-jobi* L. (Gramineae)	Refrigerant, diuretic, antirheumatic

Chinese Name (Transliteration)	Common Name	Part Used	Scientific Name (Family Name)	Medical Uses
黃 連 (Huang-lien)	Coptis	Root	*Coptis chinensis* Franch;*C. teeta* Wall. (Ranunculaceae)	Bitter stomachic, digestive, antidysenteric
山 茱 萸 (Shan-shu-yu)	Cornus	Fruit	*Cornus officinalis* Sieb. et Zucc. (Cornaceae)	Astringent tonic in impotence, spermatorrhea, lumbago, vertigo, night sweats
延 胡 索 (Yen-hu-suo)	Corydalis	Tuber	*Corydalis ambigua* Cham. et Schiecht. (Papaveraceae)	Sedative, antispasmodic, analgesic in headache, menstrual colic
津 蟹 (Chin-hsieh)	Crassipis	Body	*Eriocheir japonicus* de Haan (Grapsusae)	Dispel the pus

216

Chinese Name (Transliteration)	Common Name	Part Used	Scientific Name (Family Name)	Medical Uses
山 楂 (Shan-cha)	Crataegus	Fruit	*Crataegus pinnatifida* Bge. var. *major* N.E.Br. *C. cuneata* Sieb. et Zucc. (Rosaceae)	Digestant, antidiarrheic
巴 豆 (Pa-tou)	Croton	Seed	*Croton tiglium* L. (Euphorbiaceae)	Violent purgative in lead colic
鬱 金 (Yu-chin)	Curcuma	Rhizome	*Curcuma longa* L. (Zingiberaceae)	Aromatic stomachic, chologogue, hemostatic
菟 絲 子 (Tu-szu-tzu)	Cuscuta	Seed	*Cuscuta japonica* Choisy (Convolvulaceae)	Tonic in impotence, spermatorrhea prostatitis, neurasthenia

Chinese Name (Transliteration)	Common Name	Part Used	Scientific Name (Family Name)	Medical Uses
海螵蛸 (Hai-piao-chiao)	Cuttlebone	Back Bone	*Sepia esculenta* Hoyle (Sepiidae)	Astringent
白前 (Pai-chien)	Cynanchum	Root	*Cynanchum stauntoni* (Dcne.) Hand.-Mazz. (Asclepiadaceae)	Antitussive, expectorant
鎖陽 (Suo-yang)	Cynomorium	Stem	*Cynomorium coccineum* L. (Cynomoriaceae)	Tonic, aphrodisiac, spermatorrhea
香附 (Shiang-fu)	Cyperus	Tubercles	*Cyperus rotundus* L. (Cyperaceae)	Aromatic, stomachic, emmenagogue, sedative, analgesic

Chinese Name (Transliteration)	Common Name	Part Used	Scientific Name (Family Name)	Medical Uses
貫 眾 (Kuan-chung)	Cyrtomium	Rhizome	*Cyrtomium fortunei* J. Smith (Aspidiaceae)	Nourish the kidney, analgesic
蒲 公 英 (Pu-kung-ying)	Dandelion	Herb	*Taraxacum officinale* Weber (Compositae)	Stomachic, cholagogue, lactagogue
石 斛 (Shih-hu)	Dendrobium	Herb	*Dendrobium nobile* Lindl.; *D. sp.* (Orchidaceae)	Secretagogue, salivant, sedative
瞿 麥 (Chu-mai)	Dianthus	Herb	*Dianthus superbus* L. *D. chinensis* L. (Caryophyllaceae)	Diuretic, emmenagogue

Chinese Name (Transliteration)	Common Name	Part Used	Scientific Name (Family Name)	Medical Uses
常 山 (Charng-shan)	Dichroa	Root	*Dichroa febrifuga* Lour. (Saxifragaceae)	Antimalarial, antipyretic
鷓 鴣 菜 (Che-ku-tsai)	Digenea	Herb	*Digenea simplex* Agardh (Rhodomelaceae)	Anthelmintic
山 藥 (Shan-Yao)	Dioscorea	Root	*Dioscorea batatas* Decne (Dioscoreaceae)	Nutrient tonic, digestant in chronic enteritis, and diarrhea
續 斷 (Hsu-tuan)	Dipsacus	Root	*Dipsacus asper* Wall. (Dipsaeaceae)	Tonic, analgesic, hematic
白 扁 豆 (Pai-pien-tou)	Dolichos	Seed	*Dolichos lablab* L. (Leguminosae)	Astringent, stomachic, digestant, anthelmintic

Chinese Name (Transliteration)	Common Name	Part Used	Scientific Name (Family Name)	Medical Uses
龍　骨 (Lung-ku)	Dragon Bone	Fossilized bone	Fossilized Bones of Dinosaurs and other Reptiles	Sedative, antispasmodic, tranquilizer
骨碎補 (Ku-sui-pu)	Drynaria	Rhizome	*Drynaria fortunei* (kze.) J. Sm. (Polypodiaceae)	Nourish the kidney, hemostatic
地　龍 (Ti-lung)	Earthworm	Worm	*Allolobophora caliginosa* Trapezoides; *Pheretima asiatica* Michaelsen (Megascolecidae)	Antipyretic, bronchodilator hypotensor
旱蓮草 (鱧腸) (Han-lien-tsao)	Eclipta	Herb	*Eclipta prostrata* L. (Compositae)	Astringent hemostatic

Chinese Name (Transliteration)	Common Name	Part Used	Scientific Name (Family Name)	Medical Uses
土木香 (Tu-mu-shiang)	Elecampane	Rhizome	*Inula helenium* L. (Compositae)	Aromatic stomachic, anthelmintic, disinfectant, antiseptic, expectorant
香薷 (Shiang-ju)	Elsholtzia	Entire herb	*Elsholtzia cristata* Willd (Labiatae)	Stomachic, carminative diuretic
淫羊藿 (Yin-yang-huo)	Epimedium	Herb	*Epimedium macranthum* Moore et Decne. (Berberidaceae)	Aphrodisiac
玳瑁 (Tai-mao)	Eretmochelys	Shell	*Eretmochelys imbricata* L. (Chelonidae)	Antipyretic

Chinese Name (Transliteration)	Common Name	Part Used	Scientific Name (Family Name)	Medical Uses
枇杷葉 (Pi-pa-yeh)	Eriobotrya	Leaves	*Eriobotrya japonica* Lindl. (Rosaceae)	Antitussive, expectorant
杜仲 (Tu-chung)	Eucommia	Bark	*Eucommia ulmoides* Oliv. (Eucommiaceae)	Tonic, hypotensor with sedative and analgesic
大戟 (Ta-chi)	Euphorbia	Root	*Euphorbia pekinensis* Rupr. (Euphorbiaceae)	Purgative, diuretic
䗪蟲 (Che-chung)	Eupolyphaga	Worm body	*Eupolyphaga sinensis* W. (Corydiidae)	Expel the effused blood, treat bruise

Chinese Name (Transliteration)	Common Name	Part Used	Scientific Name (Family Name)	Medical Uses
芡 實 (Chien-shih)	Euryale	Seed	*Euryale ferox* Salisb. (Nymphaceae)	Tonic and astringent in spermatorrhea, analgesic in neuralgia, arthralgia
吳 茱 萸 (Wu-shu-yu)	Evodia	Fruit	*Evodia rutaecarpa* Bentham (Rutaceae)	Stomachic, carminative, stimulant, uterotonic
茴 香 (Hui-shiang)	Fennel	Fruit	*Foeniculum vulgare* Mill. (Umbelliferae)	Carminative, stomachic stimulant
黃 蠟 (Huang-la)	Flava Wax	Wax	*Apis chinensis* (Apidae)	Internal hemostatic, astringent

Chinese Name (Transliteration)	Common Name	Part Used	Scientific Name (Family Name)	Medical Uses
紫 石 英 (Tzu-shih-ying)	Fluorite	Mineral	CaF_2	Tranquilizer
連 翹 (Lien-chiao)	Forsythia	Fruit	*Forsythia suspensa* Vahl (Oleaceae)	Antipyretic, antiphlogistic
白 鮮 皮 (Pai-hsien-pi)	Fraxinella	Peel	*Dictamnus dasycarpus* Turcz. (Rutaceae)	Antipyretic
秦 皮 (Chin-pi)	Fraxinus	Bark	*Fraxinus rhynchophylla* Hance (Oleaceae)	Astringent, stomachic
貝 母 (Pei-mu)	Fritillaria	Bulbus	*Fritillaria verticillata* Willd.; *F. roylei* Hook. (Liliaceae)	Antitussive, expectorant in chronic trachitis, bronchitis, bronchial asthma

225

Chinese Name (Transliteration)	Common Name	Part Used	Scientific Name (Family Name)	Medical Uses
伏 龍 肝 (黃 土) (Fu-lung-kan)	Fu-Lung-Kan	Earth	The Hardened Earth found on the interior bottom of wood-burning kitchen stoves after several years of use	Sedative, antidiarrheic
(高) 良薑 (Kao-liang-chiang)	Galanga	Rhizome	*Alpinia officinarum* Hance (Zingiberaceae)	Stomachic in dyspepsia, gastralgia, chronic enteritis
釣 藤 (Kou-teng)	Gambir (Uncaria)	Spines	*Uncaria rhynchophylla* Miq. (Rubiaceae)	Sedative, antispasmodic in infantile nervous disorders
急 性 子 (Chi-hsing-tzu)	Garden Balsam	Seed	*Impatiens balsamina* L. (Balsaminaceae)	Expel the effused blood, expectorant

Chinese Name (Transliteration)	Common Name	Part Used	Scientific Name (Family Name)	Medical Uses
梔 子 (Chih-tzu)	Gardenia	Fruit	*Gardenia florida* L. *G. jasminosides* Ellis (Rutaceae)	Antipyretic, hemostatic, antiphlogistic in jaundice
天 麻 (Tien-ma)	Gastrodia	Root	*Gastrodia elata* Blume (Orchidaceae)	Tonic in vertigo, headache, myoneuralgia, rheumatism
阿 膠 (Ah-chiao)	Gelatin	Skin	*Equus asinus* L. (Equidae)	Hemostatic
接 骨 草 (Chieh-ku-tsao)	Gendarussa	Herb	*Gendarussa vulgaris* Nees (Acanthaceae)	Antirheumatism, drugs for bonesetting

Chinese Name (Transliteration)	Common Name	Part Used	Scientific Name (Family Name)	Medical Uses
芫 花 (Yuan-hua)	Genkwa	Flower	*Daphne genkwa* Sieb. et Zucc. (Thymelaeaceae)	Diuretic, stomachic, antitussive
龍 膽 (Lung-tan)	Gentiana	Root	*Gentiana scabra* Bunge (Gentianaceae)	Stomachic
生 薑 (Sheng-chiang)	Ginger	Rhizome	*Zingiber officinale* Rosc. (Zingiberaceae)	Stomachic, stimulant, antiemetic
乾 薑 (Kan-chiang)	Ginger	Rhizome	*Zingiber officinale* Rosc. (Zingiberaceae)	Stomachic, stimulant, antiemetic
白 果 (銀 杏) (Pai-kuo)	Ginkgo	Seed	*Ginkgo biloba* L. (Ginkgoaceae)	Astringent, sedative, antitussive in asthma

Chinese Name (Transliteration)	Common Name	Part Used	Scientific Name (Family Name)	Medical Uses
人 參 (Jen-sheng)	Ginseng	Root	*Panax ginseng* C.A. Meyer (Araliaceae)	Tonic, stimulant, aphrodisiac, indicated in neurasthenia, dyspepsia, palpitation, impotence, asthma
皂 角 (Tsao-chiao)	Gleditsia	Fruit	*Gleditsia sinensis* Lam. (Leguminosae)	Stimulant, expectorant
皂 刺 (Tsao-chih)	Gleditsia Spine	Stem spine	*Gleditsia sinensis* Lam. (Leguminosae)	Stimulant, expectorant
北 沙 參 (Pei-sha-sheng)	Glehnia	Root	*Glehnia littoralis* Fr. Schm. (Umbelliferae)	Expectorant, Antitussive

Chinese Name (Transliteration)	Common Name	Part Used	Scientific Name (Family Name)	Medical Uses
石 膏 (Shih-kao)	Gypsum (Gyps)	Mineral	Gypsum, Native Calcium Sulfate, Alabaster, Selenite, Satinite, Terra Alba	Sedative, antipyretic, antiphlogistic
代 赭 石 (Tai-che-shih)	Haematite	Mineral	Native Brown Iron Oxide, Fe_2O_3 and Clay	Hematonic, antiemetic, astringent, hemostatic
石 決 明 (Shih-Chueh-ming)	Haliotis (Sea-ear)	Shell	*Haliotis diversicolor* Reeve ; *H. gigantea discus* Reeve; *H. ovina* Gmelin (Haliotidae)	Sedative, alterative, hypotensor
茯 苓 (Fu-ling)	Hoelen	Fungus	*Porua cocos* Wolf. (Polyporaceae)	Diuretic, sedative, treatments of oliguresis, insomnia

Chinese Name (Transliteration)	Common Name	Part Used	Scientific Name (Family Name)	Medical Uses
蠐 螬 (Chi-tsao)	Holotrichia	Worm Body	*Holotrichia sauteri* Moser; *H. diomphallia* Bates; *Trematodes tenebrioides* Pallas (Scarabaeidae)	Expel the extravasation blood, ophthalmic
何 首 烏 (Ho-sou-wu)	Ho-Sou-Wu	Root	*Polygonum multiflorum* Thunb. (Polygonaceae)	Tonic, hematogenic
魚 腥 草 (Yu-hsing-tsao)	Houttuynia	Herb	*Houttuynia cordata* Thunb. (Saururaceae)	Diuretic, urinary antiseptic
血 餘 炭 (Hsueh-yu-Tan)	Human Hair	Hair	*Homo sapiens* (L.) (Human hair calcined and powdered) (Hominidae)	Astringent, hemostatic

231

Chinese Name (Transliteration)	Common Name	Part Used	Scientific Name (Family Name)	Medical Uses
青 黛 (Ching-tai)	Indigo	Pigment	*Indigofera tinctoria* L. (Leguminosae) *Polygonum tinctorium* (Polygonaceae)	Antiphlogistic, anticode, antipyretic
旋 覆 花 (Suan-fu-hua)	Inula	Flower	*Inula japonica* Thunb.; *I. britannica* L. (Compositae)	Expectorant, stomachic
大 棗 (Ta-tsao)	Jujube (Zizyphus)	Fruit	*Zizyphus sativa* Gaertn. (Rhamnaceae)	Nutrient tonic, sedative in insomnia, neurasthenia, mucilaginous pectoral

Chinese Name (Transliteration)	Common Name	Part Used	Scientific Name (Family Name)	Medical Uses
燈 心 草 (Teng-hsin-tsao)	Juncus	Pith	*Juncus communis* Mey.; *J. decipiens* Nakai (Juncaceae)	Diuretic, antiphlogistic
柿 蒂 (Shih-ti)	Kaki	Calyx	*Diospyros kaki* L. (Ebenaceae)	Lower the "chi", treat hiccough
甘 遂 (Kan-sui)	Kan-Sui	Root	*Euphorbia kansui* Liou (Euphorbiaceae)	Diuretic, expectorant
赤 石 脂 (Chih-shih-chih)	Kaolin	Mineral	Essentially Hydrated Aluminum Silicate	Astringent
藁 本 (Kao-pen)	Kao-Pen	Root	*Ligusticum sinense* Oliv.; *Nothosmyrnium japonicum* Miq. (Umbelliferae)	Sedative, analgesic

Chinese Name (Transliteration)	Common Name	Part Used	Scientific Name (Family Name)	Medical Uses
千 金 子 (Chien-chin-tzu)	Lathyris	Seed	*Euphorbia lathyris* L. (Euphorbiaceae)	Diuretic, expel the extravasation blood
昆 布 (Kun-pu)	Laminaria	Herb	*Laminaria japonica* Aresch. (Laminariaceae)	Alterative
馬 勃 (Ma-po)	Lasiosphaera	Fungus	*Lasiosphaera nipponica* (Kawam.) Y. Kobayashi et Y. Asahina (Lycoperaceae)	Astringent, antiphlogistic, antitussive, hemostatic
益 母 草 (I-mu-tsao)	Leonurus	Herb	*Leonurus sibiricus* L. (Labiatae)	Emmenagogue, diuretic, vasodilator

234

Chinese Name (Transliteration)	Common Name	Part Used	Scientific Name (Family Name)	Medical Uses
葶 藶 子 (Ting-li-tzu)	Lepidium	Seed	*Lepidium apetalum* Willd.; *Draba nemorosa* L. (Cruciferae)	Expectorant, diuretic
甘 草 (Kan-tsao)	Licorice	Root	*Glycyrrhiza uralensis* Fisch. (Leguminosae)	Demulcent, expectorant, emollient in peptic ulcer
女 貞 子 (Nu-chen-tzu)	Ligustrum	Fruit	*Ligustrum lucidum* Ait. *L. japonicum* Thunb. (Oleaceae)	Nutrient tonic
百 合 (Pai-ho)	Lily	Bulb	*Lilium japonicum* Thunb. (Liliaceae)	Nutrient, antitussive, expectorant

235

Chinese Name (Transliteration)	Common Name	Part Used	Scientific Name (Family Name)	Medical Uses
烏 藥 (Wu-yao)	Lindera	Root	*Lindera strychnifolia* Vill. (Lauraceae)	Aromatic, stomachic
紫 草 (紫 根) (Tzu-tsao)	Lithospermum	Root	*Lithospermum erythrorrhizon* Sieb. et Zucc. (Boraginaceae)	Antipyretic, depurative in viriola
磁 石 (Tsu-shih)	Loadstone	Mineral	Fe_3O_4, Ferrosoferric Oxide	Hematonic, sedative in tachycardia, asthma
龍 眼 肉 (Lung-yen-jou)	Longan	Aril	*Euphoria longana* (Lour.) Steud. (*Nephelium longana* Lam.) (Sapindaceae)	Nutrient tonic in neurasthenia, insomnia

236

Chinese Name (Transliteration)	Common Name	Part Used	Scientific Name (Family Name)	Medical Uses
金 銀 花 (Chin-yin-hua)	Lonicera	Flowers	*Lonicera japonica* Thunb. (Caprifoliaceae)	Diuretic, refrigerant, antiphlogistic, antidiarrheic
淡 竹 葉 (Tan-chu-yeh)	Lophatherum	Herb	*Lophatherum gracile* Brongniart (Gramineae)	Diuretic, refrigerant
桑 寄 生 (Sang-chi-sheng)	Loranthus	Entrie plant	*Loranthus parasiticus* (L.) Merr. (Loranthaceae)	Tonic, antiphlogistic, hypotensor
蓮 房 (Lien-fang)	Lotus Peduncle	Peduncle	*Nelumbo nucifera* Gaertn. (Nymphaceae)	Hemostatic
蓮 子 (Lien-tzu)	Lotus Seed	Seed	*Nelumbo nucifera* Gaertn. (Nymphaceae)	Tonic, diarrhea

237

Chinese Name (Transliteration)	Common Name	Part Used	Scientific Name (Family Name)	Medical Uses
蓮 鬚 (Lien-hsu)	Lotus Stamens	Stamens	*Nelumbo nucifera* Gaertn. (Nymphaceae)	Astringent
水 燈 香 (Shui-teng-shiang)	Ludwigia	Root & stem	*Ludwigia octovalvis* (Jacq.) Raven (Onagraceae)	Antipyretic, diuretic
枸 杞 子 (Kou-chi-tzu)	Lycium Fruit	Fruit	*Lycium chinense* Mill. (Solanaceae)	Nutrient tonic in diabetes, mellitus, pulmonary tuberculosis
地 骨 皮 (Ti-ku-pi)	Lycium Bark	Root epidermis	*Lycium chinense* Mill. (Solanaceae)	Antipyretic, antitussive in pulmonary tuberculosis

Chinese Name (Transliteration)	Common Name	Part Used	Scientific Name (Family Name)	Medical Uses
伸 筋 草 (Sheng-chin-tsao)	Lycopodium	Herb	*Lycopodium clavatum* (Lycopodiaceae)	Carminative, improve the blood circulation, analgesic
海 金 沙 (Hai-chin-sha)	Lygodium	Spore	*Lygodium japonicum* (Thunb.) Sw. (Schizaeceae)	Antiphlogistic, diuretic, dysuria
茜 草 (Chien-tsao)	Madder	Root	*Rubia cordifolia* L. (Rubiaceae)	Emmenagogue, hemostatic
厚 朴 (Hou-pu)	Magnolia Bark	Bark	*Magnolia officinalis* Reh. et Wils. (Magnoliaceae)	Antispasmodic, stomachic, antiseptic

Chinese Name (Transliteration)	Common Name	Part Used	Scientific Name (Family Name)	Medical Uses
辛夷 (Hsin-i)	Magnolia Flower	Flower	*Magnolia liliflora* Desr. (Magnoliaceae)	Tonic, analgesic in sinusitis, rhinitis, coryza, headache, vertigo
麻黃 (Ma-huang)	Ma-Huang	Stem	*Ephedra sinica* Stapf (Ephedraceae)	Bronchial asthma, hay fever, trachitis
麥芽 (Mai-ya)	Malt	Fruit	*Hordeum vulgare* L. (Gramineae)	Stomachic, digestant
膠飴 (Chiao-i)	Maltose	Fruit	*Oryza sativa* L. *Triticum aestivum* L. (Gramineae)	Tonic

Chinese Name (Transliteration)	Common Name	Part Used	Scientific Name (Family Name)	Medical Uses
桑 螵 蛸 (Sang-piao-chiao)	Mantis	Chrysalis	*Paratenodera sinensis* de Saussure; *Mantis religiosa* L. (Mantidae)	Nourish the kidney, tonic in impotence, spermatorrhea, enuresis
乳 香 (Ju-shiang)	Mastic	Resin	*Pistacia lentiscus* L. *Boswellia glabra* (Anacardiaceae)	Analgesic, sedative, as antitussive, expectorant
蜂 蜜 (Feng-mi)	Mel (Honey)	Honey	*Apis cerana* Fabr. *A. chinensis* (Apidae)	Astringent, demulcent, diarrheic, analgesic
綠 礬 (Lu-fan)	Melanterite	Mineral	Green Vitriol, Ferrous Sulfate, $FeSO_4 \cdot 7H_2O$	Astringent, hematonic

241

Chinese Name (Transliteration)	Common Name	Part Used	Scientific Name (Family Name)	Medical Uses
苦 楝 子 (Ku-lien-tzu)	Melia	Fruit	*Melia toosendan* S. et Z. *M. azedarach* L. (Meliaceae)	Anthelmintic
苦 楝 皮 (Ku-lien-pi)	Melia Bark	Bark	*Melia toosendan* S. et Z. *M. azedarach* L. (Meliaceae)	Anthelmintic
甜 瓜 蒂 (Tien-kua-ti)	Melo Pedicel	Pedicel	*Cucumis melo* L. (Cucurbitaceae)	Expectorant, emetic
薄 荷 (Po-ho)	Mentha	Leaves	*Mentha arvensis* L. var. *piperascens* Malinv. (Labiatae)	Stomachic, carminative, stimulant, diaphoretic

Chinese Name (Transliteration)	Common Name	Part Used	Scientific Name (Family Name)	Medical Uses
雞 血 藤 (Chi-hsueh-teng)	Millettia	Stem	*Millettia reticulata* Benth. (Leguminosae)	Tonic, prevail the meridians
鉛 丹 (Chien-tan)	Minium	Mineral	Red Lead Oxide, Pb_3O_4	Externally as disinfectant, antiphlogistic in conjuctivitis, cuts, and burns
芒 硝 (Mang-hsiao)	Mirabilitum	Mineral	Mirabilitum	Cathartic, diuretic
巴 戟 天 (Pa-chi-tien)	Morinda	Root	*Morinda officinalis* How (Rubiaceae)	Impotence, antirheumatic

243

Chinese Name (Transliteration)	Common Name	Part Used	Scientific Name (Family Name)	Medical Uses
桑 白 皮 (Sang-pai-pi)	Morus	Root epidermis	*Morus alba* L. (Moraceae)	Antitussive, expectorant in asthma, bronchitis, cough
桑 枝 (Sang-chih)	Morus Branch	Branch	*Morus alba* L. (Moraceae)	Anti-rheumatism, diuretic
桑 椹 (Sang-chen)	Morus Fruit	Fruit	*Morus alba* L. (Moraceae)	Tonic
桑 葉 (Sang-yeh)	Morus Leaves (Mulberry Leaves)	Leaves	*Morus alba* L. (Moraceae)	Influenza, headache
木 鼈 子 (Mu-pieh-tzu)	Momordica	Seed	*Momordica cochinchinensis* Spreng.(Cucurbitaceae)	Dispel the swelling, detoxifier

244

Chinese Name (Transliteration)	Common Name	Part Used	Scientific Name (Family Name)	Medical Uses
牡 丹 皮 (Mu-tan-pi)	Moutan	Root bark	*Paeonia moutan* Sims (Ranunculaceae)	Antipyretic, emmenagogue, for infectious of the digestive tract
烏 梅 (Wu-mei)	Mume	Unripe fruit	*Prunus mume* Sieb. et Zucc. (Rosaceae)	Stomachic, antipyretic, astringent
麝 香 (She-shiang)	Musk	Secretion	*Moschus moschiferus* L. (Dried secretion from preputial follicles of the Musk-Deer) (Cervidae)	Cardiotonic, stimulant
沒 藥 (Mo-yao)	Myrrh	Resin	*Commiphora myrrha* Engler (Burseraceae)	Exsiccant, stomachic, antispasmodic

Chinese Name (Transliteration)	Common Name	Part Used	Scientific Name (Family Name)	Medical Uses
川 骨 (Chuan-ku)	Nuphar	Root	*Nuphar japonica* DC. (Nymphaceae)	Hemostatic, astringent
五 倍 子 (Wu-pei-tzu)	Nutgalls	Galls	*Rhus chinensis* Miller (*R. semialata* Murray) (Anacardiaceae)	Astringent, styptic
反 鼻 (Fan-pi)	Ophidia	Body	*Trigonocephalis blomhoffi* Boie (Gotalidae)	Tonic, dispel the pus
麥 門 冬 (Mai-men-tong)	Ophiopogon	Root	*Ophiopogon japonicus Liriope spicata* Lour. (Liliaceae)	Antitussive, expectorant, emollient, antiscrifulous

Chinese Name (Transliteration)	Common Name	Part Used	Scientific Name (Family Name)	Medical Uses
橘 紅 (Chu-hung)	Orange Peel	Exocarp	*Citrus reticulata* Blanco (Rutaceae)	Expectorant
粳 米 (Keng-mi)	Oryza	Seed	*Oryza sativa* L. (Gramineae)	Tonic, stomachic
牡 蠣 (Mu-li)	Ostrea Testa (Oyster Shell)	Shell	*Ostrea gigas* Thunb.; *O. talienwhanensis* Crosse; *O. rivularis* Gould (Ostreidae)	In hyperchlorlydria
赤 芍 (芍 藥) (Chih-shao)	Paeonia	Root	*Paeonia lactiflora* Pall. *P. albiflora* Pall. (Ranunculaceae)	Gastric disorders, as intestinal antiseptic, expectorant, emmenagogue

Chinese Name (Transliteration)	Common Name	Part Used	Scientific Name (Family Name)	Medical Uses
白 薇 (Pai-wei)	Pai-Wei	Root	*Cynanchum atratum* Bge. (Asclepiadaceae)	Diuretic, antipyretic
真 珠 (Chen-chu)	Pearl	Pearl	*Pteria margaritifera* (L.);*P. martensii* Dunker (Pteriidae) *Cristaria plicata* Leech (Unionidae)	Sedative in insommia, headache, convulsions
紫 蘇 葉 (Tzu-su-yeh)	Perilla	Leaves	*Perilla fructescens* Britt. (Labiatae)	Antitussive, stomachic, antiseptic
紫 蘇 子 (Tzu-su-tzu)	Perilla Seed	Seed	*Perilla fructescens* Britt. (Labiatae)	Antitussive, stomachic, antiseptic

248

Chinese Name (Transliteration)	Common Name	Part Used	Scientific Name (Family Name)	Medical Uses
桃 仁 (Tao-jen)	Persica	Seed	*Prunus persica* (L.) Batsch (Rosaceae)	Antitussive, sedative in hypertension
前 胡 (Chien-hu)	Peucedanum	Root	*Peucedanum decursivum* Max. (Umbelliferae)	Analgesic, antipyretic, expectorant
牽 牛 子 (Chien-niu-tzu)	Pharbitis	Seed	*Ipomoea hederacea* Jacq. (*Pharbitis hederacea* Choisy) (Convolvulaceae)	Cathartic, diuretic, anthelmintic
赤 小 豆 (Chih-hsiao-tou)	Phaseolus	Seed	*Phaseolus calcaratus* Roxb. (Leguminosae)	Diuretic, dispel the effused blood, antipyretic, detoxifier

249

Chinese Name (Transliteration)	Common Name	Part Used	Scientific Name (Family Name)	Medical Uses
黃蘗 (Huang-po)	Phellodendron	Bark	*Phellodendron amurense* Rupr. (Rutaceae)	Stomachic, antiseptic, externally as antiphlogistic in skin diseases
蘆根 (Lu-ken)	Phragmites	Rhizome	*Phragmites communis* Trin. (Gramineae)	Stomachic, antiemetic, antipyretic
葦莖 (Wei-ching)	Phragmites stem	Stem	*Phragmites communis* Trin. (Gramineae)	Stomachic, antiemetic, antipyretic
商陸 (Shang-lu)	Phytolacca (Pokeberry)	Root	*Phytolacca esculenta* Vanh; *P. acinosa* Roxb. (Phytolaccaceae)	Diuretic

250

Chinese Name (Transliteration)	Common Name	Part Used	Scientific Name (Family Name)	Medical Uses
半 夏 (Pan-hsia)	Pinellia	Tuber	*Pinellia tuberifera* Breitenbach (Araceae)	Antiemetic, sedative, antitussive in nausea, pharyngalgia, singultus, chronic gastritis
油 松 節 (Yu-sung-chieh)	Pinus Node	Wood	*Pinus tabulaeformis* Carr.; *P. massoniana* Lamb. (Pinaceae)	Carminative, demulcent
松 香 (松 脂) (Sung-shiang)	Pinus Resin	Resin	*Pinus massoniana* Lamb. (Pinaceae)	Analgesic, stimulant, dispel the pus, diuretic hemostatic (external)
蓽 茇 (Pi-pa)	Piper (Long Pepper)	Fruit	*Piper longum* L. (Piperaceae)	Aromatic, stomachic, analgesic

Chinese Name (Transliteration)	Common Name	Part Used	Scientific Name (Family Name)	Medical Uses
紫 河 車 (Tzu-ho-che)	Placenta	Placenta	*Homo sapiens* L. (Hominidae)	In impotence, neurasthenia, infecundity
車 前 子 (Che-chien-tzu)	Plantago	Seed	*Plantago asiatica* L. (Plantaginaceae)	Diuretic, expectorant
桔 梗 (Ciiie-keng)	Platycodon	Root	*Platycodon grandiflorum* A. DC. (Campanulaceae)	Expectorant
遠 志 (Yuan-chih)	Polygala	Root	*Polygala tenuifolia* Willd. (Polygalaceae)	Expectorant, cardiotonic, renal tonic
玉 竹 (Yu-chu)	Polygonatum	Rhizome	*Polygonatum canaliculatum; P. officinale* All. (Liliaceae)	Tonic

Chinese Name (Transliteration)	Common Name	Part Used	Scientific Name (Family Name)	Medical Uses
萹 蓄 (Pien-hsu)	Polygonum	Herb	*Polygonum aviculare* L. (Polygonaceae)	Diuretic, anthelmintic, antidiarrheic, antiphlogistic
豬 苓 (Chu-ling)	Polyporus	Fungus	*Grifola umbellata* Pilat. (Polyporaceae)	Arrests locd, hemorrhages
眞 珠 母 (Chen-chu-mu)	Pteria	Shell	*Pteria martensii* Dunker (Pteridae); *Hyriopsis cumingii* Lea (Unionidae)	Hemostatic
夏 枯 草 (Hsia-ku-tsao)	Prunella	Inflorescence	*Prunella vulgaris* L. (Labiatae)	Alterative, antipyretic, diuretic in scrofula, gout

Chinese Name (Transliteration)	Common Name	Part Used	Scientific Name (Family Name)	Medical Uses
三 七 (San-chi)	Pseudoginseng	Root	*Panax pseudoginseng* Wall.(Araliaceae)	Hemostatic, analgesic
補 骨 脂 （破故紙） (Pu-ku-chih)	Psoralea	Seed	*Psoralea corylifolia* L. (Leguminosae)	Tonic, stimulant
五 靈 脂 (Wu-ling-chih)	Pterpous	Excrement	*Pteropus pselaphon* Lay (Pteropodidae)	Analgesic, emmena-gogue
葛 根 (Ko-ken)	Pueraria	Root	*Pueraria thunbergiana* Benth.; *P. pseudo-hirsuta* Tang et Wang (Leguminosae)	Antipyretic, refrigerant

254

Chinese Name (Transliteration)	Common Name	Part Used	Scientific Name (Family Name)	Medical Uses
葛 花 (Ko-hua)	Pueraria Flower	Flower	*Pueraria thunbergiana* Benth;*P. pseudohirsuta* Tang et Wang (Leguminosae)	Antipyretic, refrigerant
浮 石 (海浮石) (Fu-shih)	Pumice	Mineral	Mainly Complex Silicates of Aluminum, Sodium, Potassium	Sedative, alterative, expectorant
石 韋 (Shih-wei)	Pyrrosia	Herb	*Pyrrosia sheareri* (Bak.) Ching; *P. petiolosa* (Christ) Ching (Polypodiaceae)	Diuretic, antigonorrhoic, expel the moisture and fever
羌 活 (Chiang-huo)	Qianghuo	Rhizome	*Notopterygium sp.* (Umbelliferae)	Diaphoretic

255

Chinese Name (Transliteration)	Common Name	Part Used	Scientific Name (Family Name)	Medical Uses
使 君 子 (Shih-chun-tzu)	Quisqualis	Fruit	*Quisqualis indica* L. (Combretaceae)	Vermifuge
兩 頭 尖 (Liang-tou-chien)	Raddeana	Rhizome	*Anemone raddeana* Regel (Ranunculaceae)	Used for cold, expectorant
萊 菔 子 (Lai-fu-tzu)	Raphanus	Seed	*Raphanus sativus* L. (Cruciferae)	Stomachic, expectorant
雄 黃 (Hsiung-huang)	Realger	Mineral	As_2S_2	Astringent, anthelmintic detoxifier

256

Chinese Name (Transliteration)	Common Name	Part Used	Scientific Name (Family Name)	Medical Uses
地 黃 (Ti-huang)	Rehmannia	Rhizome	*Rehmannia glutinosa* Libosch. (Scrophulariaceae)	Cardiotonic, diuretic, hemostatic in diabetes mellitus
犀 角 (Hsi-chiao)	Rhinoceros	Horn	*Rhinoceros unicornis* L. *R. sondaicus* Desmarest *R. sumatrensis* Cuvier (Rhinocerotidae)	Antipyretic, cool the blood, detoxifier
大 黃 (Ta-huang)	Rhubarb	Rhizome	*Rheum palmatum* L. *R. officinale* Baill. (Polygonaceae)	Stomachic in gastric, catarrh and diarrhea
金 櫻 子 (Chin-ying-tzu)	Rosa Fruit	Fruit	*Rosa laevigata* Michx. (Rosaceae)	Carminative, astringent tonic

Chinese Name (Transliteration)	Common Name	Part Used	Scientific Name (Family Name)	Medical Uses
覆 盆 子 (Fu-pen-tzu)	Rubus	Fruit	*Rubus chingii* Hu; *R. coreanus* Miq. (Rosaceae)	Astringent
番 紅 花 (Fan-hung-hua)	Saffron	Stigm	*Crocus sativus* L. (Iridaceae)	Improve the circulation, antipyretic
丹 参 (Tan-sheng)	Salvia Root	Root	*Salvia miltiorrhiza* Bunge (Labiatae)	Female tonic in amenorrhea, metrorrhagia, gastralgia, mastitis
硝 石 (Hsiao-shih)	Saltpeter	Mineral	KNO_3	Demulcent

258

Chinese Name (Transliteration)	Common Name	Part Used	Scientific Name (Family Name)	Medical Uses
檀 香 （檀 木） (Tan-shiang)	Santalum	Wood	*Santalum album* L. (Santalaceae)	Aromatic stomachic, carminative, analgesic in nervous gastralgia
蘇 木 (Su-mu)	Sappan-Wood	Wood	*Caesalpinia sappan* L. (Leguminosae)	Hemostatic, astringent
海 藻 (Hai-tsao)	Sargassum	Herb	*Sargassum fusiforme* (Harv.) Setch. (Sargassaceae)	Diuretic. used for iodine deficiencies
紅 藤 （大血藤） (Hung-teng)	Sargentodoxa	Stem	*Sargentodoxa cuneata* (Oliv.) Rehd. et Wils. (Sargentodoxaceae)	Carminative, prevail the veins & meridians, diuretic, anthelmintic

259

Chinese Name (Transliteration)	Common Name	Part Used	Scientific Name (Family Name)	Medical Uses
木 香 (Mu-shiang)	Saussurea	Root	*Saussurea lappa* Clarke (Compositae)	Treatment of asthma, stomachic
五 味 子 (Wu-wei-tzu)	Schizandra	Fruit	*Schizandra chinensis* Baillon (Magnoliaceae)	Tonic, stimulant, antitussive
荆 芥 (Ching-chieh)	Schizonepeta	Whole herb	*Schizonepeta tenuifolia* Briq. (Labiatae)	Diaphoretic, antipyretic
三 稜 (San-leng)	Scirpus	Rhizome	*Scirpus martimus* L. (Cyperaceae)*Sparganium romosum* Huds. (Sparganiaceae)	Emmenagogue, analgesic, laxative
全 蠍 (Chuan-hsieh)	Scorpion	Worm body	*Buthus martensi* Karsch (Buthidae)	Antispasmodic, nerve tonic

260

Chinese Name (Transliteration)	Common Name	Part Used	Scientific Name (Family Name)	Medical Uses
玄 參 （元 參） (Hsuan-tsan)	Scrophularia	Root	*Scrophularia ningpoensis* Hemsley (Scrophulariaceae)	Cardiotonic, as antipyretic, antiphlogistic
黃 芩 (Huang-chin)	Scute	Root	*Scutellaria baicalensis* Georgi (Labiatae)	Stomachic, antipyretic, expectorant
小 薊 (Hsiao-chi)	Segetum	Herb	*Cirsium segetum* Bge. (Compositae)	Dispel the effused blood, cool the blood, hemostatic
胡 麻 子 (Hu-ma-tzu)	Sesame	Seed	*Sesamum indicum* L. (Pedaliaceae) *Linum usitatissimum* L. (Linaceae)	As lenitive in scybalous constipation; as nutrient tonic in degenerative neuritis, neuroparalysis

261

Chinese Name (Transliteration)	Common Name	Part Used	Scientific Name (Family Name)	Medical Uses
栗 米 (Su-mi)	Setaria	Seed	*Setaria italica* (L.) Beauv. (Gramineae)	Nourish the spleen, digestive, stomachic
紫 鉚 (Tzu-kwang)	Shellac	Lac	The resinous excretion from the female *Laccifer lacca* on the tree, esp. at the ends of branches while it lives on	Antipyretic, detoxifier
神 麯 (Shen-chu)	Shen-Chu	Preparation	*Xanthium strumarium* L.; *Artemisia apiacea* Hance; *Phaseolus celcaratus* Roxb. etc.	Digestant

262

Chinese Name (Transliteration)	Common Name	Part Used	Scientific Name (Family Name)	Medical Uses
豨 莶 草 (Hsi-chien-tsao)	Siegesbeckia	Herb	*Siegesbeckia pubescens* Mak.; *S. orientalis* L. (Compositae)	Analgesic, antirheumatic
防 風 (Fang-Feng)	Siler	Root	*Siler divaricatum* Benth. et Hook.; *Ledebouriella seseloides* Wolff. (Umbelliferae)	Antipyretic, analgesic
殭 蠶 (Chiang-tsan)	Silk-worm	Worm	*Bombyx mori* L. (Bombycidae)	Sedative, analgesic, expectorant
土 茯 苓 (Tu-fu-ling)	Smilax	Root	*Smilax china* L. *S. glabra* Roxb. (Liliaceae)	Alterative, diuretic in syphilis, gout, skin disorders, rheumatism

Chinese Name (Transliteration)	Common Name	Part Used	Scientific Name (Family Name)	Medical Uses
（淡）豆豉 (Tan-tou-shih)	Soja	Preparation	*Glycine max* (L.) Merr. (Leguminosae)	Antipyretic
苦 参 (Ku-sheng)	Sophora	Root	*Sophora flavescens* Ait. (Leguminosae)	Bitter stomachic astringent in dysentery, enterorrhagia
八角茴香 (Pa-chiao-hui-shiang)	Star Anise	Fruit	*Illicium verum* Hook. (Magnoliaceae)	Stomachic, stimulant
百 部 (Pai-pu)	Stemona	Root	*Stemona sessilifolia* (Miq.) Franch. et Savat.; *S. tuberosa* Lour. (Stemonaceae)	Antitussive, pediculicide

264

Chinese Name (Transliteration)	Common Name	Part Used	Scientific Name (Family Name)	Medical Uses
防 己 (Fang-chi)	Stephania	Root	*Stephania* tetrandra S. Moore (Menisper-maceae)	Antipyretic, diuretic, analgesic, arthritis, lumbago, myalgia
蘇 合 香 (Su-ho-shiang)	Styrax	Resin	*Liquidambar orientalis* Miller (Hamanelidaceae)	Stimulant, expecto-rant
琥 珀 (Hu-po)	Succinum	Resin	The resinous exudate from plants of pina-ceous pine species, which has been buried underground for a long time and became clear, fossil-like substance.	Aphrodisiac, anthelmintic

Chinese Name (Transliteration)	Common Name	Part Used	Scientific Name (Family Name)	Medical Uses
硫 黃 (Liu-huang)	Sulfur	Mineral	The innate sulfur after a preliminary processing	Vermicide, laxative
蝱 蟲 (Mang-chung)	Tabanus (Gadfly)	worm	*Tabanus mandarinus* Schi.;*T. bovinui* (Tabanidae)	Emmenagogue
滑 石 (Hua-shih)	Talc	Mineral	Native Hydrous Magnesium Silicate, $3MgO \cdot 4SiO_2 \cdot H_2O$	Antiphlogistic, hemostatic, diuretic
當 歸 (Tang-kuei)	Tang-Kuei	Root	*Angelica sinensis* Diels (Umbelliferae)	Emmenagogue, sedative, analgesic

266

Chinese Name (Transliteration)	Common Name	Part Used	Scientific Name (Family Name)	Medical Uses
黨 參 (Tang-sheng)	Tang-Sheng	Root	*Codonopsis tangshen* Oliver (Campanulaceae)	Tonic in anemia, chronic enteritis, gastricatony
細 茶 (Hsi-cha)	Tea	Leaves	*Thea sinensis* L. *(Camellia sinensis* Kuntze) (Theaceae)	Cardiotonic, central nerve stimulant, diuretic, intestinal astringent
訶 子 (Ho-tzu)	Terminalia	Fruit	*Terminalia chebula* Retz. (Combretaceae)	Astringent, hemostatic, antidiarrhea, antitussive
通 草 (Tung-tsao)	Tetrapanax	Pith	*Tetrapanax papyrifera* (Hook) K. Koch (Araliaceae)	Diuretic, galactagogue

Chinese Name (Transliteration)	Common Name	Part Used	Scientific Name (Family Name)	Medical Uses
敗 醬 (Pai-chiang)	Thlaspi	Herb	*Thlaspi arvense* L. (Cruciferae) *Patrinia scabiosaefolia* Link. (Valerianaceae)	Antipyretic, detoxifier, improve the circulation, dispel the pus, expectorant, diaphoretic
虎 骨 (虎脛骨) (Hu-ching-ku)	Tiger's Shinbone	Bone	*Panthera tigris* L. (*Felis tigeris*). (Felidae)	Analgesic, strengthen the bone and muscle, sedative
蟾蜍 (Tsan-yu)	Toad	Body	*Bufo bufo gargrizans* Cantor; *Bufo melanostictus* Schneider (Bufonidae)	Expel the moisture & fever, dispel the swelling, analgesic, detoxifier

Chinese Name (Transliteration)	Common Name	Part Used	Scientific Name (Family Name)	Medical Uses
蟾 酥 (Tsan-shu)	Toad Secretion	Secretion	*Bufo bufo gargarizans* Cantor; *Bufo melanostictus* Schneider (Bufonidae)	Detoxifier, analgesic, tonic, diuretic
萆 薢 (Pi-hsieh)	Tokoro	Root	*Dioscorea sativa* L. *D. tokoro* Makino (Dioscorea)	Diuretic
鱉 甲 (Pieh-chia)	Tortoise Shell	Carapace	*Amyda sinensis* (Trionychidae)	Antipyretic, tonic
菱 角 (Ling-chueh)	Trapa	Fruit	*Trapa natans* L. (Trapaceae)	Tonic, antipyretic

Chinese Name (Transliteration)	Common Name	Part Used	Scientific Name (Family Name)	Medical Uses
蒺 藜 (Ciu-li)	Tribulus	Fruit	*Tribulus terrestris* L. (Zygophyllaceae)	Tonic, astringent
栝 樓 根 (Kua-lou)	Trichosanthes Root	Root	*Trichosanthes kirilowii* Max. (Cucurbitaceae)	Antipyretic
栝 樓 子 (栝樓仁) (Kua-lou-tzu)	Trichosanthes Seed	Seed	*Trichosanthes kirilowii* Max. (Cucurbitaceae)	Antitussive, expectorant as emollient for skin swellings
草 果 (Tsao-kuo)	Tsao-Ko	Fruit	*Amomum tsao-ko* Crevost et Lem. (Zingiberaceae)	Digestive, expectorant

270

Chinese Name (Transliteration)	Common Name	Part Used	Scientific Name (Family Name)	Medical Uses
草 豆 蔻 (Tsao-tou-kou)	Tsao-Tou-Kou	Seed	*Alpinia katsumadai* Hay. (Zingiberaceae)	stomachic
獨 活 (Tu-huo)	Tuhuo	Root	*Angelica laxiflora* Diels *A. grosseserrata* Maxim. (Umbelliferae)	Antispasmodic, analgesic, diaphoretic, diuretic
薑 黃 (Chiang-huang)	Turmeric	Rhizome	*Curcuma aromatica* Salisb. (Zingiberaceae)	Dispel the effused blood, emmenagogue, analgesic
龜 板 (Kuei-pan)	Turtle Shell	Carapace	*Chinemys reevesii* (Gray) (Testudinidae)	Nutrient tonic

Chinese Name (Transliteration)	Common Name	Part Used	Scientific Name (Family Name)	Medical Uses
款 冬 花 (Kuan-tong-hua)	Tussilago	Floral buds	*Tussilago farfara* L. (Compositae)	Antitussive, expectorant
蒲 灰 (Pu-huei)	Typha Ash	Leaves	*Typha angustata* Bory et Chaub; *T. latifolia* L. (Typhaceae)	Diuretic
王不留行 (Wang-pu-liu-hsing)	Vaccaria	Seed	*Vaccaria pyramidata* Medic.(Caryophyllaceae)	Emmenagogue, analgesic
槲 寄 生 (Hu-chi-seng)	Viscum	Entire plant	*Viscum album* L. (Loranthaceae)	Hypotensor, lactagogue, antiphlogistic

Chinese Name (Transliteration)	Common Name	Part Used	Scientific Name (Family Name)	Medical Uses
蔓 荊 子 (Mian-ching-tzu)	Vitex	Fruit	*Vitex rotundifolia* L. *V. trifolia* L. (Verbenaceae)	Sedative, analgesic
浮 小 麥 (Fu-hsiao-mai)	Wheat	Fruit	*Triticum aestivum* L. (Gramineae)	Sedative, antipyretic
紫 藤 瘤 (Tzu-teng-liu)	Wistaria	Gall	*Wistaria floribunda* D.C. (Leguminosae)	Stomachic, antiphlogistic
烏 頭 (Wu-tou)	Wu-Tou	Root	*Aconite carmichaeli* Debx. (Ranunculaceae)	Antispasmodic, sedative, analgesic
蒼 耳 子 (Tsang-erh-tzu)	Xanthium	Fruit	*Xanthium strumarium* L. (Compositae)	Antipyretic, antispasmodic, diaphoretic

Chinese Name (Transliteration)	Common Name	Part Used	Scientific Name (Family Name)	Medical Uses
川 椒 (花 椒) (Chuan-chiao)	Zanthoxylum	Fruit	*Zanthoxylum piperitum* DC.; *Z. simulans* Hance (Rutaceae)	Stimulant, tonic, stomachic, carminative, diuretic
椒 目 (Chiao-mu)	Zanthoxylum Seed	Seed	*Zanthoxylum simulans* Hance (Rutaceae)	Diuretic, drugs for edema & swelling
烏 梢 蛇 (Wu-shao-sheh)	Zaocys	Body	*Zaocys dhumnades* Contor (Colubridae)	Antispasmodic, carminative
莪 朮 (O-chu)	Zedoaria	Rhizome	*Curcuma zedoaria* Rosc. (Zingiberaceae)	Dispel the stagnant blood, smooth the "chi", digestant

Chinese Name (Transliteration)	Common Name	Part Used	Scientific Name (Family Name)	Medical Uses
酸 棗 仁 (Suan-tsao-jen)	Zizyphus (Jujuba)	Seed	*Zizyphus jujube* Mill. *Z. sativa* var. *spinosa* (Rhamnaceae)	Nutrient tonic, sedative, insomnia, neurasthenia

FORMULA INDEX

A

Almond and Cannabis Formula (76)*
Areca Combination (8)
Areca and Evodia Combination (110)
Astragalus Combination (87)
Atractylodes Combination (92)

B

Bamboo and Hoelen Combination (122)
Minor Blue Dragon Combination (18)
Bupleurum and Cinnamon Combination (59)
Bupleurum and Dragon-Bone Combination (62)
Bupleurum and Hoelen Combination (114)
Bupleurum and Peony Formula (36)
Bupleurum and Pueraria Combination (61)
Bupleurum and Schizonepeta Formula (1)
Bupleurum and Scute Combination (115)

C

Capillaris Combination (69)
Capillaris and Hoelen Five Formula (65)
Cardamon and Fennel Formula (41)
Chrysanthemum Combination (97)
Cimicifuga Combination (1)

G

Gasping Formula (108)
Gentiana Combination (105)
Ginseng and Astragalus Combination (96)
Ginseng and Atractylodes Formula (82)
Ginseng and Ginger Combination (2)
Ginseng and Gypsum Combination (29)

---

* number of Formula from Page 48 - 100

Z

CHINESE CROSS-REFERENCE
OF FORMULAS

A

An-Chung-San
(Cardamon and Fennel Formula)

安中散 [41]

An-Tai-Yin
(Tang-Kuei and Parsley Combination)

安胎飲 [57]

C

Chai-Hsien-Tang
(Bupleurum and Scute Combination)

柴陷湯 [115]

**Chai-Hu-Chia-Lung-Ku-
Mu-Li-Tang**
(Bupleurum and Dragon-Bone Combination)

柴胡加龍骨牡蠣湯 [62]

**Chai-Hu-Kuei-Chih-Kan-
Chiang-Tang**
(Bupleurum, Cinnamon, and Ginger Combination)

柴胡桂枝乾薑湯 [60]

Chai-Hu-Kuei-Chih-Tang
(Bupleurum and Cinnamon Combination)

柴胡桂枝湯 [59]

Chai-Ko-Chiai-Chi-Tang
(Bupleurum and Pueraria Combination)

柴葛解肌湯 [61]

Chai-Ling-Tang
(Bupleurum and Hoelen Combination)

柴苓湯 [114]

Chen-Wu-Tang
(Vitality Combination)

眞武湯 [63]

Chi-Li-San
(Musk and Catechu Formula)

七厘散 [111]

I

I-Kan-San
(Bupleurum Formula) 抑肝散 [45]

I-Tzu-Tang
(Tang-Kuci and Bupleurum Combination) 乙字湯 [1]

I-Yi-Jen-Tang
(Coix Combination) 薏苡仁湯 [106]

J

Jen-Sheng-Pai-Tu-San
(Ginseng and Mentha Formula) 人參敗毒散 [4]

Jen-Sheng-Tang
(Ginseng and Ginger Combination) 人參湯 [2]

Jen-Sheng-Tang-Shao-San
(Ginseng and Tang-Kuei Formula) 人參當芍散

Jen-Sheng-Yang-Yung-Tang
(Ginseng Nutritive Combination) 人參養榮湯 [3]

K

Kan-Lu-Yin
(Sweet Combination) 甘露飲 [40]

Kan-Mai-Ta-Tsao-Tang
(Licorice and Jujube Combination) 甘麥大棗湯 [38]

Kan-Tsao-Fu-Tzu-Tang
(Licorice and Aconite Combination) 甘草附子湯

Kan-Tsao-Hsieh-Hsin-Tang
(Pinellia and Licorice Combination) 甘草瀉心湯 [39]

W

Selected Bibliography

I. ENGLISH SOURCES

Hsu Hong-yen and Peacher, William. *Chinese Herb Medicine and Therapy*. Los Angeles: Oriental Healing Arts Institute, 1976.

Hsu Hong-yen and Peacher, William. *Chen's History of Chinese Medicine*. Los Angeles: Oriental Healing Arts Institute, 1977.

Hsu Hong-yen. *Chinese Herbs and Formulas*. Los Angeles: Oriental Healing Arts Institute, 1978.

II. CHINESE SOURCES

Hsu Hong-yen. *Chung-yao cheng-fen tsui-chin yen-chiu* (Recent Advances in the Study of Chinese Herbal Medicine). Taipei: Kuo-li chung-kuo i-hsueh yen-chiu-suo, 1968.

Hsu Hong-yen. *Chang yung chung-yao chih yen-chiu* (A Study of Commonly Used Chinese Herbal Formulas). Taipei: Hsin-cheng-yuan wei-sheng-shu chung-i-yao-yuan-hui, 1972.

Hsu Hong-yen. *Chung-kuo i-yao kai-nien* (A General View of Chinese Medicine). Taipei: Hsin-cheng-yuan wei-sheng-shu chung-i-yao-yuan-hui, 1973.

Hsu Hong-yen. *Shao yung chung-yao chih yen-chiu* (A Study of Seldom Used Chinese Herbal Formulas). Taipei: Hsin-cheng-yuan wei-sheng-shu chung-i-yao-yuan-hui, 1974.

Hsu Hong-yen. *Chung-yao cheng-fen chih hua-hsueh* (The Chemical Makeup of Chinese Herbal Medicine Constituents). Taipei: Hsin-cheng-yuan wei-sheng-shu chung-i-yao-yuan-hui 1975.

Hsu Hong-yen. *K'uang-wu hsing chung-yao yen-chiu* (A Study of Chinese Mineral Drugs). Taipei: Kuo-li chung-kuo i-yao yen-chiu-suo, 1975.

Hsu Hong-yen. *Tzu-chien tzu-liao* (Self Treatment and Self Healing). Taipei: Hsin i-yao chu-pan-she, 1977.

Hsu Hong-yen. *Chung-i pien-cheng kang-yao* (The Essentials of Confirmation in Chinese Medicine). Taipei: Hsin i-yao chou-kan she, 1977.

Hsu Hong-yen. *Tung-wu hsing chung-yao chih yen-chiu* (A Study of Chinese Animal Drugs). Taipei: Kuo-li chung-kuo i-yao yen-chiu-suo, 1977.

Hsu Hong-yen. *Han-fang tui i-nan cheng chih chih-liao* (Chinese Herbal Medicine and its Treatment of Degenerative Diseases). 2 vols. Taipei: Hsin i-yao chu-pan-she, 1979.

Hsu Hong-yen. *Chien-kang chieh-ching* (The Way to Health and Happiness). Taipei: Hsin i-yao chu-pan-she, 1979.

Otsuka, Keisetsu et al. *Han-fang chen liao i-tien* (A Dictionary of Diagnosis and Treatment in Chinese Medicine). Taipei: Kuo-li chung-kuo i-yao yen-chiu-suo, 1973.

III. JAPANESE SOURCES

Isihara, Akira. *Kanpō* (Chinese Medicine). Tokyo: Chion-kouranshia, 1967.

Otsuka, Keisetsu ed. *Kanpō daijiten* (A Dictionary of Chinese Medicine). Tokyo: Koutanshia, 1975.

Otsuka, Keisetsu ed. *Kanpō, harikyu: kate chiriyo* (Self Treatment with Chinese Medicine and Acupuncture). Tokyo: Hokendouzinsha, 1976.

Terashi, Bokusa. *Kanpō no shindan chiriyo* (Diagnosis and Treatment in Chinese Medicine). Tokyo: Fukumura, 1976.